ADVANCE PRAISE

As the 'Momma of VBAC' I wasn't sure what to expect when I opened Ilia Blandina's book; I took a breath and hoped there would be something of value inside. It's wonderful. It is filled with excellent information for how to achieve a natural birth after having had a c-section. Ilia 'gets it' - that how a woman births and how a baby is born is *extremely* important. She gives women hope as well as practical suggestions. She makes sense. I called her as soon as I finished reading and thanked her, as her book fills my heart with hope. Ilia is, indeed, one of my VBAC daughters!

–NANCY WAINER, CPM
THE PIONEERING MIDWIFE WHO COINED THE TERM "VBAC".
SHE IS THE AUTHOR OF *SILENT KNIFE: CESAREAN PREVENTION
AND VBAC; OPEN SEASON: A SURVIVAL GUIDE FOR NATURAL
BIRTH* AND THE SOON TO BE RELEASED *BIRTHQUAKE: A PRE-
AND POST CHILDBIRTH BOOK FOR STRONG WOMEN AND WOMEN
WHO WANT TO BE STRONG*

*****

Full disclosure: I am Ilia's husband, and the father of all four of her sons. Our sons. To say that this book was a labor of love for Ilia, is not really accurate. It was a driving passion of hers to get this information into the hands of as many pregnant or planning to be pregnant, women as possible.

Even though I am not really a part of her intended audience, I am a part of her story, and I share her desire to have as many people get in touch with their bodies, and have information that can make people feel confident in the natural function of their body.

T0163599

I think the book is highly readable, yet blends spirituality and science seamlessly. I have always felt that the most spiritual moments in my life were being there for the birth of our four sons.

I highly recommend this book for everyone, including expectant dads. It is chock full of insight to the wonderful gift of childbirth.

–GARY BLANDINA
AUTISM COACH, SPECIAL EDUCATION TEACHER

*****

In many Western cultures, especially in the U.S., there is much fear and many misconceptions about having a vaginal birth after C-section. Traditional allopathic doctors in the field are taught to direct and control what should be a natural process, often disregarding a mother's needs, wants and desires. Because medical practices now are based primarily upon a model of risk management, women's rights and choices have been pushed to the sidelines. This has led to the birth crisis we see today where C-section rates continue to rise at astronomical rate.

Ilia Blandina's book, *Give Birth a Chance: How to Prepare for an Empowered VBAC*, not only gives that choice back to women but also does it in such a way that women can have a thoroughly educated and informed choice to have the birth they've always wanted. Given that Ilia Blandina worked extensively as a nurse midwife professionally and then faced her own VBAC, the material in this book will inspire you to take action, create a plan, and calm the voices of fear that surround the decision to have a vaginal birth after having had a C-section. The author packs this book full of invaluable exercises that will guide the reader step-by-step. We will be using it as a resource for anyone we know that is looking for answers to a topic that is wrought with misinformation and fear-based approaches.

–CRAIG WEINER AND ALINA FRANK
EMOTIONAL FREEDOM TECHNIQUES (EFT) INTERNATIONAL
TRAINERS, AUTHOR OF THE BEST-SELLING *HOW TO WANT SEX
AGAIN: REKINDLING PASSION WITH EFT*

Give Birth A Chance gives the reader so much more than information and knowledge about how to have an empowered VBAC. It is written by a midwife and mother who has experienced personally having a VBAC and also experienced what is going on in the 'medical world' and allows the reader to make powerful and informed choices. She provides techniques and practical exercises and ways of preparing for birth which can be used by first time mothers-to-be as well. So well researched and so much experience to be gained from reading this book and from the 'toolkit' provided. If you want to have an empowered VBAC or a powerful birth, then this is the book for you!

–JENNY JOHNSTON
FOUNDER OF QUANTUM EFT. EFT TRAINER AND
BEST-SELLING AUTHOR OF *TAPPING INTO PAST LIVES*.
WWW.QUANTUMEFT.COM.AU

*****

It's hard to believe that a new book about childbirth can possibly have new information to offer. But here it is. *Give Birth A Chance* is a delightfully refreshing, very complete guide to successful birthing – for any woman. You don't have to be wanting a VBAC, or having your first baby to benefit from the information and recommendations gathered here. I am proud of Ilia for the message she conveys and the courage to express the truth. As a provider of out-of-hospital birth services, I intend to make this book required reading for all of my clients.

–P. FADWAH HALABY
CNM, FOUNDER & OWNER OF MIDWIFE360,
SPECIALIZING IN HOMEBIRTH

Give Birth a Chance empowers women seeking vaginal birth after cesarean and brings light to the many shortfalls of hospitals in maternity care and labor/delivery. I have long said that the media is responsible for creating fear during delivery. You have to watch a documentary on natural child birth to see a peaceful birth these days. I especially love the positive affirmations and the many exercises that Ilia includes to change your perception on pain. This book is not only great for educating one on vaginal birth after cesarean, it is great for anyone who is pregnant and fears delivery.

–CANDISS O'REILLY
CO-OWNER AT ECO BABY EXPO

*****

Ilia Blandina's book, *Give Birth A Chance*, surprised me. What I thought was going to be a book focused on having a vaginal birth after a cesarean (VBAC) is a comprehensive guide to having an empowering birth experience for the mother, her partner, and baby. She goes into great detail about the history, science, and nature of birth covering how the mind and body work together while giving tips on how to achieve the birth you desire. I highly recommend this book to any pregnant woman who wants an empowering birth.

–KERRY MARRAFFINO
MOM & CROSSFITTER,
HTTP://KERRYMARRAFFINO.COM/

Ilia Blandina's book, *Give Birth A Chance: How to Prepare for an Empowered VABC*, guides readers through the miracle that is birth, aids in our re-membering of ancestral birth wisdom, and provides an honest assessment of current healthcare practices with regard to vaginal birth after C-section (VBAC). Her book provides a workable roadmap for VBAC success, introducing Emotional Freedom Techniques (EFT) concepts. With strategies for easy application during pregnancy and labor, her book is an appropriate resource for both the novice and seasoned practitioner supporting mothers seeking a VBAC or preparing for the birth process in general.

–NIKKI SMITH-ROMAIN
MSN, LCCE DOULA, CHILDBIRTH EDUCATOR
WWW.MIDWIFE360.COM

*****

Give Birth A Chance is a MUST read for all who are considering becoming pregnant as well as parents considering adding to their family and I would like to add, future grandparents.

Though I had my babies in the '70's I learned some valuable information which I will share with my clients, family and friends and definitely encourage them to read *Give Birth A Chance*, by Ilia Blandina.

Personally, I loved being pregnant and for me the deliveries were like having bad cramps. As I was reading, memories did return of how our doctor had us sign papers to release him and the hospital from all liabilities because I refused all drugs. My first pregnancy was during the return of 'natural' childbirth and the Lamaze breathing technique.

A couple years later we chose to have our baby at home. Again, as Ilia describes in her book, the best laid birth plan doesn't necessarily work out as planned. I intuitively listened to my body and knew I had to head to the hospital. Fortunately, we were able to still deliver our baby using the Laboyer Method. No drugs and the atmosphere was calming, dimmed lights and warm.

I feel our experience was positive even though it was in the hospital because I was able to research doctors and our new doctor was a gem. He was very willing to allow our baby to arrive in his own time.

I do get upset reading about the increase in C-sections being performed mainly for convenience and not caring for the parents and the baby's experience.

Ilia is an expert in her field. If you have questions and or fears I highly recommend her as your go to expert.

You are very fortunate to have this great resource at your figure tips.

Embrace your birth journey, do your due-diligence and ultimately trust and listen to your body.

–SANDY CONCAR
INTUITIVE AND INTEGRATIVE HEALTH,
WWW.BALANCELIFENATURALLY.COM

GIVE BIRTH A CHANCE

GIVE BIRTH A CHANCE

How to Prepare for an
Empowered VBAC

BY ILIA BLANDINA, CNM

NEW YORK

LONDON • NASHVILLE • MELBOURNE • VANCOUVER

GIVE BIRTH A CHANCE

How to Prepare for an Empowered VBAC

Published in New York, New York, by Morgan James Publishing in partnership with Difference Press. Morgan James is a trademark of Morgan James, LLC. www.MorganJamesPublishing.com

The Morgan James Speakers Group can bring authors to your live event. For more information or to book an event visit The Morgan James Speakers Group at www.TheMorganJamesSpeakersGroup.com.

This book does not provide medical advice, professional diagnosis, opinion, treatment, or services. Any medical advice quoted by the author in this book is paraphrased and/or quoted and should not reflect on the actual advice given by your personal healthcare providers. The author of this book is providing general and anecdotal information for educational purposes only. All medical decisions should be discussed and made together with your healthcare providers.

This book depicts actual events in the life of the author as truthfully as recollection permits and/or can be verified by research. Occasionally, dialogue consistent with the character or nature of the person speaking has been supplemented. All persons within may be actual individuals or composite characters. The names of individuals have been changed to respect their privacy.

ISBN 9781683505198 paperback
ISBN 9781683505204 eBook
Library of Congress Control Number: 2017905175

Cover Design by:
Doreen Hann

Author Photo courtesy of:
The Picture Producer, LLC

Interior Design by:
Chris Treccani
www.3dogcreative.net

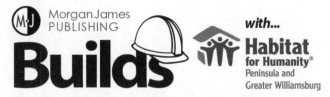

In an effort to support local communities, raise awareness and funds, Morgan James Publishing donates a percentage of all book sales for the life of each book to Habitat for Humanity Peninsula and Greater Williamsburg.

Get involved today! Visit
www.MorganJamesBuilds.com

DEDICATION

For Gary, Alex, Andrew, Aaron, and Adam,
my greatest teachers of love, birth, and life.

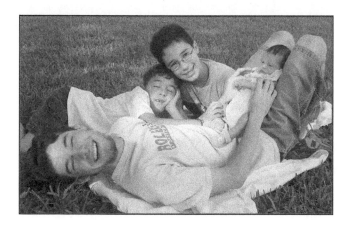

TABLE OF CONTENTS

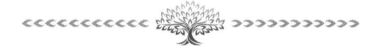

FOREWORD

Give Birth A Chance: How to Prepare for an Empowered VBAC is a guide to childbirth for our times. Ilia Blandina has captured one of the most pressing concerns for women giving birth today: the climbing rate of cesarean sections. Vaginal birth after cesarean or C-section (VBAC) has been slowly removed as a choice for many healthy, low risk women. This has caused increased long term risks for both mother and baby, which are well covered throughout the book.

Ilia brings to you an experienced look at the pitfalls and solutions to your search for an empowered birth experience based on her firsthand knowledge of obstetric health care, having been a certified nurse midwife (CNM) for 25 years in various settings and having cared directly for over 5000 women in childbirth.

This book will not only help a cesarean section mama prepare for an empowered VBAC, it is also a fantastic guide for first time moms and dads to prepare for birth and avoid an unnecessary C-section all together. Ilia's mission to help mothers, fathers and partners prepare for the birth of their dreams is evident throughout this incredible guide. I was honored to be introduced to Ilia by Karen Brody founder of the BOLD movement and playwright of *Birth*. After talking with Ilia and reading the book I instantly knew that our missions for improving childbirth through respectful, pleasurable, evidenced based birth were in complete alignment.

I myself understand what it is like to be a pioneer in reminding humanity that birth can be full of pleasure and delight. I have trained thousands of doulas and birth professionals around the world in the practices of gentle birth support. I also created and directed *Orgasmic Birth: The Best-Kept Secret*, a documentary examining the intimate nature of birth, an everyday miracle. What Ilia and I have in common is seeing the powerful role birth plays in women's lives when they are permitted to experience it fully. Having also co-authored the book *Orgasmic Birth: Your Guide to a Safe, Satisfying and Pleasurable Birth Experience*, I understand the importance of getting as much evidenced-based childbirth education out to the people who are in contact with expecting families, as well as expectant families themselves.

Ilia has blended her expertise in helping women give birth from her many firsthand experiences as a CNM and now with her Emotional Freedom Techniques (EFT) practice to bring women new and innovative exercises to neutralize any fears or doubts about the birth process. In doing so, Ilia has created a new path towards experiencing an empowered, gentle and intimate birth journey. If you are not yet familiar with EFT, Ilia will guide you through the basics of EFT and then ways to use it during pregnancy and childbirth preparation.

This book also addresses many of the pitfalls of modern obstetric care in the United States today. With a focus on the model of risk management, obstetrics is slowly eroding the women's rights of childbirth choices, including the right to choose a VBAC. These practices are what led to the childbirth crisis we see today where C-section rates are 32% nationally and can reach as high as 68% for an individual hospital. Ilia, through her book, has brought to light much of the fear and misconceptions about having a VBAC. Not only has she helped women with these fears as a CNM, but she herself was faced with her own VBAC. All of these experiences inspired her to write this invaluable book full of exercises and step-by-step guidance for helping expectant families looking for answers to a healthcare crisis that is full of misinformation and fear-based approaches.

Ilia has also incorporated the concepts of looking towards our ancestors for guidance, creating an awareness of the higher self and the importance of maintaining the sacred power of birth itself. For women wanting to create a birth plan, Ilia teaches how to create a personalized plan that not only taps into what you want your birth to be like but also connects you with the power of intention during your planning in order to create an empowered birth journey.

Ilia ends the book with a fantastic view of the future of birth, creating a *Give Birth A Chance Manifesto* and inviting you as the reader and recipient of the legacy to join in on its planning. I highly recommend you read this book. I have found Ilia's unique storytelling and guidance in *Give Birth A Chance* to be an outstanding resource of guidance to awaken your intuitive wisdom as it empowers women, their families and communities towards healthy birth choices and preparation for empowered births.

DEBRA PASCALI-BONARO, B.ED., LCCE, PDT/BDT(DONA)
FOUNDER & PRESIDENT OF PAIN TO POWER CHILDBIRTH
EXPERIENCE, DIRECTOR OF THE AWARD-WINNING
DOCUMENTARY *ORGASMIC BIRTH: THE BEST-KEPT SECRET*

JANUARY 3, 2017
RIVER VALE, NJ

PREFACE

The universe has led you to find this book for a reason. If you are really committed to having a vaginal birth after cesarean (VBAC), this is your first step. The ability to be able to choose VBAC as a birth option has personally and professionally affected me. I am a midwife passionate about helping women overcome their fears and doubts when they are planning their birth. I have blended my skills as a Certified Nurse Midwife (CNM) and Emotional Freedom Techniques (EFT) practitioner to empower women during pregnancy and when giving birth.

This book is meant to be the beginning of our conversation. In it, you will find some harsh realities we face as women while we go forth and prepare for childbirth. I decided to focus on the importance of preparing for VBAC because of the wildly increasing cesarean section rate in our country and in the world at large. The same concepts and principles can be applied if this is your first birth, and will prepare you to avoid having a cesarean section (aka C-section or section) in the first place.

Wouldn't it be grand and beautiful if the need for this book becomes extinct, as opposed to our ability of giving vaginal birth becoming extinct? The protection of vaginal birth needs to be paramount in order to protect humanity as a whole. You will come to this conclusion as well after reading this book.

ILIA BLANDINA, CNM
September 10, 2016
Florida

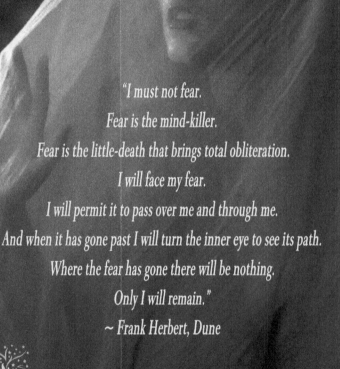

"I must not fear.

Fear is the mind-killer.

Fear is the little-death that brings total obliteration.

I will face my fear.

I will permit it to pass over me and through me.

And when it has gone past I will turn the inner eye to see its path.

Where the fear has gone there will be nothing.

Only I will remain."

~ Frank Herbert, Dune

INTRODUCTION

"You've thrown the worst fear that can ever be hurled.
Fear to bring children into the world.
For threatening my baby, unborn and unnamed,
you ain't worth the blood that runs in your veins."
~**BOB DYLAN**, *MASTERS OF WAR*

It's Okay to Want a VBAC

t seems like wanting to have a vaginal birth after cesarean (VBAC) is such a taboo these days! It doesn't have to be this way. But this whole thing of being afraid for the life of your baby is so powerful; it almost makes you want to throw in the towel before you even get started.

I am here to let you know that you don't have to feel alienated when you bring up the subject of VBAC with your practitioner, friends, or family. You have a choice. Don't let yourself be talked out of a VBAC, also known as trial of labor after a cesarean section (TOLAC). You might feel alone in this decision, but you are not.

Your first baby may have been born via a C-section, and now you are starting to think maybe it's time for her or him to have a brother or sister. It's taken you a while to consider trying to have a baby again because your first birth didn't go as planned – in fact, it was awful. You felt that

xxviii | GIVE BIRTH A CHANCE

you weren't given enough time to labor at your own pace. You really wanted a natural birth but it seemed like no one listened, and instead it all snowballed into everything you didn't want to happen, happening.

Labor started at home but after arriving at the hospital, you slowly realized your progress was being measured against someone else's formulated schedule out of a text book with no regard to how your body responds to labor. You were pronounced "slow" because you didn't meet up with mainstream medicine's time constraints. One thing led to the next, and before you knew it, you were somehow late to your own baby's birth. Suddenly, in the middle of trying to deal with your pain from the contractions, someone on the delivery team was telling you that you needed a cesarean section.

Today, years afterwards, you are a working mom and you want to have your next baby. This might be your last childbirth, but you're not sure. The one thing you *are* sure of is that you do not want it to go like the first birth. You still don't really understand what went wrong and why you ended up with a C-section. Your baby was born healthy, and you were fine except for having a slow labor.

How do you make sure things go differently the next time around? After all, you thought you had it all under control the first time. You went to childbirth education classes, you read all "the right books," you got your husband involved; you wrote out a birth plan, you had a great midwife and doula. You really thought you did everything right.

The ultimate fear of going for a trial of labor after cesarean (TOLAC) is that your uterine incision will break open. This risk has been overstated and is actually very low. It has been used as the main reason to talk women into repeat C-sections without really going into true informed consent. The reality is that a VBAC has lower risks than a repeat C-section, and I will be going over this in detail later in the book.

The Curse of the Birth Plan

What you may not have known during your last pregnancy is the "curse of the birth plan." Part superstition and part sad truth, it basically means that birth plans generally get thrown out the window – not because of their existence, but because of the way they are worded. In Chapter 3, I will teach you how to write the perfect individualized birth plan that will energetically put you in alignment with what you want your birth journey to look like.

Since you didn't have your dream birth the first time, it's understandable to worry that you won't be able to do it next time, either. And most mainstream medicine practitioners support that fear. No matter how you slice it (no pun intended), you carry the stigma of having had a C-section.

They will say "you don't have a proven pelvis." This statement means that since you have not had a vaginal delivery before, no one knows how well you will do in labor. But this is true of any first-time moms and is usually not mentioned to them. In essence, the message being given is that "your body can't be trusted with a vaginal birth." Reading blogs about how the statement "proven pelvis" is received by most expectant moms has been very enlightening. Some women have even changed healthcare providers after this terminology was used because they felt misunderstood, misguided, and prejudged.

You've probably already learned it's hard to find a practitioner who is not rooted in fear-based, liability-avoidance delivery practices. In other words, it will be hard to find someone willing to help you with a VBAC. You may have found out that the hospital and doctor you thought would be there for you are really out for themselves. They have their own agenda, and they are carrying out that agenda according to policies and procedures under the pretense of it being in your best interest. Unfortunately, you find out if you don't fall in line with what they "require," they will not help you get the birth you want, long for, and is safer for you.

All you know is that you want that dream vaginal birth of your ancestors. The one that shows you are an empowered woman, giver of life, over comer of obstacles. The one who has complete trust in her body, connecting with the stars, planets, and universe through an experience that no one should ever take away just because it doesn't fit into their "time frame."

It's Okay to Be Angry

When you think about your first birth, you are angry that you didn't stand your ground – and yet you also feel guilty, ashamed, and embarrassed. You may be asking yourself, "Was it too much to expect to have a normal birth the first time around?" Your baby is healthy. How can you overcome all these mixed feelings? Should you just give in and schedule your repeat cesarean section like everyone is telling you to do? After all, you can pick the date of delivery, no waiting, no stress.

NO! You want to have the birth of your dreams! You don't care if you have to say, "Fuck you!" to the establishment.

On the other hand, you really want to be as ready as possible. You realize that acknowledging your own fears and doubts so that you can attract the right people and resources into your life is very important. You want to be a strong warrior goddess during your next birth.

So far, all you are sure of is that this time you want to take charge and be as informed as you can be. You want to get a handle on all your fears and doubts. You want to not only be proactive in your decision-making process, but also know how to be proactive during labor. You want nothing to get in the way of you and your empowered birth. You don't want to be misinformed again.

But from the beginning, you are feeling like you are being set up to doubt yourself, your decision, and your body. During the very first visit, your practitioner starts to make you feel like you are putting your baby's life at risk for even considering a VBAC. Then, during one of your many sleepless nights, you are searching the internet for information and you find horror stories about doctors who have gotten court orders for women to have a repeat cesarean section.

You know this is rare, but the fact it happens makes shivers run up your spine. You start to wonder; how can I avoid this? How can I surround myself with what I need and the people who will support me to meet my needs? How do I overcome the bias of a fearful medical community? In your desperation, you Googled "How do I plan a VBAC?" You find this book, and here we are, face to face.

The Mental Struggle for a VBAC Is Real

After going through a successful VBAC, I'm here to tell you it doesn't have to be so complicated. Although at the time, planning my VBAC sure *seemed* complicated. Since I am a midwife, my peers thought I should know better and just have a repeat C-section. I should be fully aware of the risks and not want to put myself or my baby in harm's way. My colleagues were all telling me I shouldn't be willing to take any risk at all.

Except that I knew deep down that having a repeat C-section actually carried more risk, and my gut feeling was later proved correct in the research of today. I was pregnant with my last baby after having had a C-section with my third. By the time I was 30 weeks pregnant, I couldn't take it anymore. I felt like I was in a war zone: Battlefield Birth!

Think about it. Here I am, a well-educated and experienced midwife, and all of the nurses I work with in labor and delivery keep telling me I will be risking my life and my baby's life. It was hell to have colleagues in the industry questioning my belief in myself and my body. And so if it was such a struggle for me as an insider, I can imagine that for someone who does not work in the healthcare industry, it must seem insurmountable. I see you out there in the struggle of wanting a VBAC but not being able to find the support you need to make it happen.

I believe that our civil rights as women to have a vaginal birth have been slowly eroded by fear. The limitations imposed on our birth options are fueled by our fear as expectant moms of whether we can do it, practitioners' fear of being sued, and hospitals' fear of being rated unsafe due to increased liability. Hospitals are always struggling for financial survival and for control of their practitioners (i.e., doctors and midwives) by being perpetual Monday morning quarterbacks. I have nothing against peer review procedures, but when they are combined with policies to increase revenue by imposing unnecessary policies and procedures, that's where I draw the line.

In essence, the medical system has stripped away women's abilities to trust their bodies. Is it a patriarchal control and convenience scheme disguised as "keeping everyone safe"? I believe it is, and I have had this happen in my own personal birth experiences.

Professionally, I know the struggle because it was very difficult to find a practice to work for where the doctors were in agreement about offering VBACs to their clients. Personally, I've been in your shoes and I found that it was a struggle to make my own VBAC happen – and I am "an insider"!

I have had four baby boys. I was very lucky with my first baby because I had found – way in advance of becoming pregnant – a doctor and midwife team that really believed in a woman's ability to give birth. They believed in natural birth so much that they even had a birth center in their office. In 1988, my doctor had a 12% C-section rate, which was difficult to find back then and almost nonexistent today.

Here is what I was personally up against during my first labor:

- The baby was three weeks overdue.
- Labor lasted over three days.

- He was in a posterior position (the back of his head was against my tail bone – which is the hardest and longest labor to have).
- I stalled out at 7 cm at the birth center for five hours. (I had to be transferred for Pitocin augmentation of labor in the hospital.)
- It took three more hours to get to 10 cm and start pushing after an epidural and Pitocin.
- I was exhausted and pushing was ineffective.

In today's birth climate, any of the reasons listed above would have been enough to force me to get a C-section. But I chose my doctor wisely, and baby Alexander was born vaginally with a little help from my doc using a vacuum assist.

My second delivery was also vaginal. I still didn't get my birth center birth; I had to be transferred to the hospital because they thought he had pooped inside. Nevertheless, I studied and figured out how to avoid back labor and baby Andrew came after only being in labor for 18 hours! (This was much better than three days.) I will cover how to avoid back labor later in the book.

Baby Aaron gave me a whole different experience. Everything went well; I had chosen to have my best friend, who happened to be a midwife, take care of me. She only did hospital births and I had moved 350 miles away from the birth center where I tried to give birth during my first two pregnancies. I thought it would be fairly easy; it was my third pregnancy.

It was a very fast labor, about six hours, but surprise! He was breech, and I was 8 to 9 cm with a strong urge to push. Unfortunately, my midwife's back-up doctor did not do breech deliveries and I had to have a C-section!

In 2003, I lived in Broward County, Florida, and I was pregnant with my last baby. The cesarean section rate was starting to climb, while the VBAC rate was in decline. I had taken a hiatus from midwifery and was a labor floor nurse again. I did manage to find a doctor willing to do a VBAC, but my colleagues, in their attempts to show concern for me, continually questioned my decision to have a VBAC.

Advice ranged from "Are you sure you want to do this?" to "You and your baby could die." I would answer back, "What's it to you, this is my body and my life. I trust my body." However, my resolve began to erode inconspicuously.

I started to buy into the idea of having a hospital birth, handpicking my anesthesiologist for my epidural, handpicking my labor nurse. After all I had the advantage of being an "insider."

I thought I had made up my mind, until the day when I was happily talking about my birth plan at the front desk with the other nurses and receiving kudos for a plan well laid out. A midwife colleague strongly said, "You don't need all of that! You should know better, trust your body, you've done this before. Don't let anyone inject their fear into you and deprive you of the birth you really want and deserve." She literally rang my bell; I awakened from the slumber of letting other peoples' fears control me.

Later, at home, I found myself alone, feeling like I was in an abyss, a war zone of mistrust: Battlefield Birth again! No support anywhere to be seen or felt. Yes, my husband Gary supported me, but he was busy working and had no inside connection.

How could I make my birth dream come true, once and for all? Did I have to run away and live in a distant land where women believe in the power of their body? Who could I talk to? Of course! Other midwives, people who innately understand my language and where I am coming from.

First, I called my friend where I studied midwifery; she was surprised that I even picked a doctor to care for me in the first place. I told her that he was all I could find because of the VBAC issue, even though I had delivered two previous babies vaginally without a problem. She offered to transfer my care to her and move in during the last month of my pregnancy as a last resort. Midwives are so wonderful; I'm so glad I am a midwife!

Ok, that was one option, but it would have been too disruptive for my family. I thought about it and then remembered my friend who was a midwife specializing in home births. I called her, told her my dilemma, and could not hold back the tears. I felt defeated, trapped, no way out of this fear-based VBAC wasteland. She said to come over right away; she wanted to do some acupuncture to help with my stress and fear-based thinking.

We talked, and Gary came to be with us after work. She gently said, "Well you know, this is your fourth baby and you want to stay home as long as possible, so maybe it might be a good idea to be ready for a home birth." She was great, she made it clear that nothing had to be written in stone, let's just see what happens, "keep seeing your doctor and we'll take it one week at a time."

Time passed, I felt emotionally supported and I had time to work through all my fears and doubts. When the big day came, everything was in place. I had all the things I needed and the comfort of home and the people I loved surrounding me with their support.

It was the most empowering experience I've ever had. My labor started at 6:30 pm and became very active by 10:30 pm, just in time for my oldest son to arrive home after the high school football game. He became the photographer of the birth and my friend who had picked him up from the school was the videographer.

I had planned for a water birth, but when it came time I couldn't stand to be in the tub. I made my way to the bed and Adam came shortly after midnight, right on his due date; all my other babies were late, but he was on time. To this day, I remember my husband whispering in my ear, "You did it! You found your Holy Grail! You can stop searching now." That moment was so powerful that now, 13 years later, I am still committed to helping woman find their "Holy Grail" of birth.

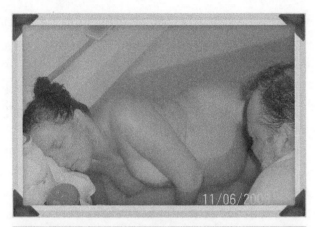

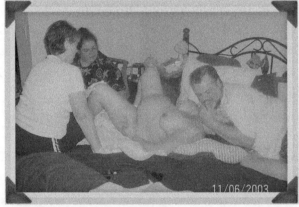

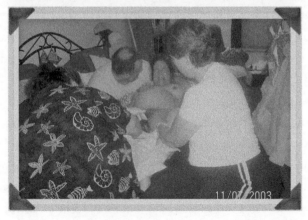

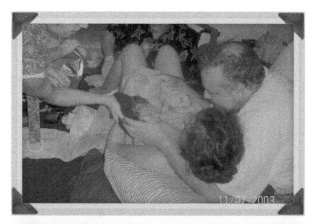

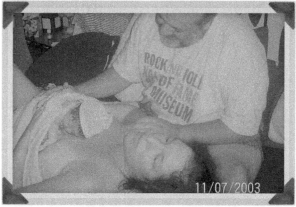

A powerful moment and realization that I did it!

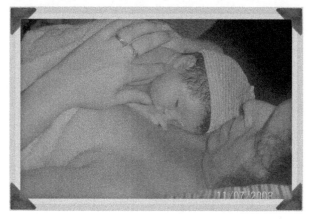

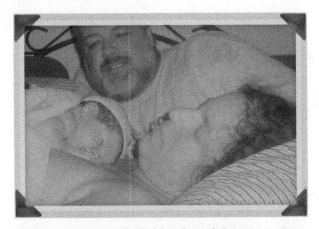

My wonderful husband Gary!

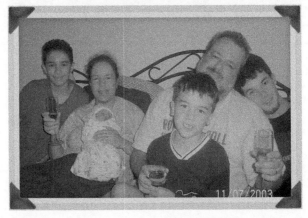

A toast to a dream fulfilled!

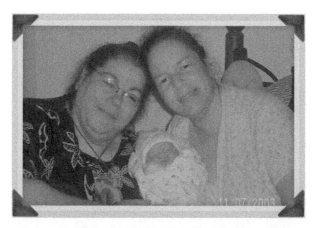

Janice, my wonderful midwife.

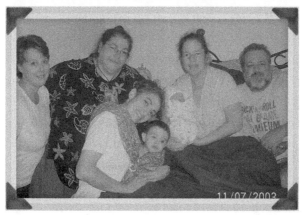

The midwife team!

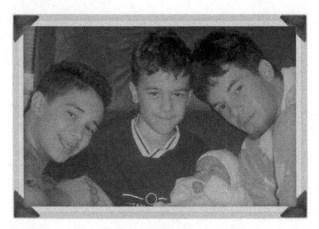

The Boyz! My four winds ♥

After that birth, I returned to being a midwife helping women deliver at local hospitals, but my heart was slowly breaking because of the rise in the cesarean section rates and the fear-based thinking of my colleagues. When my body said "no" to any more deliveries and endless nights on call, I decided it was time to help women get their dream birth in an unique way and that is what this book is all about.

Having a VBAC delivery with my last pregnancy was a bit of a struggle even for someone in the business. But the bottom line was that Baby Adam was born at home and was the "Holy Grail" of birth I always was searching for. I want you to know that if you really want a VBAC, it can happen. And I want to share with you how you can empower your own birth journey and trust your deepest desire.

I've been collecting information, studying, and practicing these techniques with my client's birth preparations and for my own births. Now that I am retired from physically delivering babies, I thought it would be a good time to share this information so that more women can benefit in the years to come.

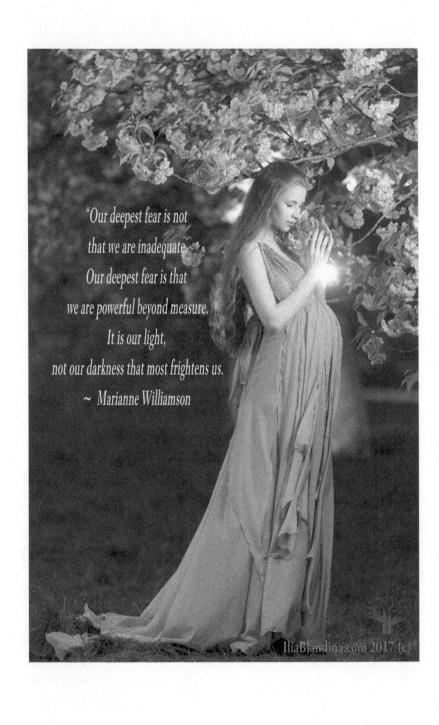

"Our deepest fear is not
that we are inadequate.
Our deepest fear is that
we are powerful beyond measure.
It is our light,
not our darkness that most frightens us.
~ Marianne Williamson

IliaBlandina.com 2017 (c)

CHAPTER 1

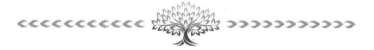

Our Ancestors

"Cut not the wings of your dreams,
for they are the heartbeat and freedom of your soul."
~FLAVIA

Only If You Want a VBAC

I am not here to talk you into something you don't already want to do. If you think this book is going to *convince* you to have a vaginal birth after cesarean section (VBAC), know that is not my intent. But if you want a VBAC, this book can give you the information you need to help you discuss your options with your healthcare practitioner.

This book is for the woman that knows deep down in her heart that she should have had a vaginal birth to begin with and somehow a cascade of interventions happened that led her away from a vaginal birth and into a C-section instead. If this is you, welcome! You have found the path towards your search for the Holy Grail of birth on your own terms and free from the negative emotional garbage of the past.

You have found our ancestors' path, the one that was taken away from us with the advent of the modern birth machine. We as woman need to get back to our roots in order to save the normal birth process before we lose all the wise women traditional knowledge.

We have lost sight of our heritage through the advent of modern obstetrics and technology. In service of keeping birth "safe," we as women have been led to believe that an environment of medical intervention, intense vigilance, and blocking the sensations of birth is a safer one in which to give birth.

In essence, we have been led far away from the truth – and we are losing the art of giving birth as a species as a result. If we don't stop the modern birth machine dynamics and give vaginal birth a chance, we are at great risk of endangering humanity as a whole.

These are strong words, which I will explain later in the book. But for right now, I want you to contemplate the many thousands of generations of mothers that have gone through the natural birth process to make it possible for you to even exist.

You may be saying, "Well, my mother needed a C-section and so did her mother. What are you talking about?" Think about it: way before them, you have grandmothers of grandmothers of grandmothers that gave birth in their communities surrounded by other women who also did the same. They all survived, or you would not be here now.

Let's Visit Our Ancestors

Let's go back in time and relive what it would have been like to give birth as it was intended from the beginning of time on planet Earth, also known by the ancient peoples as Gaia. The spirit of Earth is Gaia, it's meant to support us, and has done so for as long as humans have existed.

Yes, our bodies were intentionally designed to give birth gracefully and in our own unique way.

Picture a community living by the sea or river, where most tribes lived for ease of access to water and food. Whether a seaside village, forest or jungle, each tribe had their council of elders. These elders were women.

The women were the wisdom keepers for the village and carried the knowledge of their ancestors, the Grandmothers. These were the women who taught the way of community life, healing, and birth; they were the way keepers, the healers, and the midwives. They had years of expertise in the art of guiding women through their birth journeys.

Our ancestral journey through life started as maidens: young, beautiful, carefree, learning the beginning of the way keepers and helping the families, healers, and midwives of the village.

As we grew, we learned about how to gather food and herbs. We learned how to make teas and salves for healing. The boys and men were busy hunting and keeping the village safe from predators as we chatted and chased after our children.

In fact, our biology, both male and female, was uniquely designed for this cooperative community. While hunting, the men had to learn to stay quiet and focused in order to follow their prey from behind bushes or trees. So, in their most stressed environment, they naturally became quiet and went inward until it was time to take action and pounce on their hunt.

You may recognize this type of behavior today in your male partner. It's in his biology to become quiet and still and to retreat when stress is at its highest. It makes sense that the modern male retreats into video games of hunting and battle.

Let's go back to the village of our ancestors. The women are gathered around the fire, cooking, caring for babies and toddlers, breastfeeding, chatting away about the tasks at hand, maybe even planning rites of passage for women who are now pregnant: the rite of passage to motherhood with all its mysteries and magic.

The sounds of all the chatter by the fire at the heart of the community are full of laughter. The more excited and energized the women and children become, the louder and more talkative they are. In some magical form of communication, they talk with each other by overlapping beginnings and ends of sentences, almost like a continuous hum of singsong harmony.

Back then, women felt heard and were always sought after for advice. The wonderful thing about all this energetic and joyful noise is that, when combined with fire, it keeps animal predators away from the village, creating a sound and light barrier of safety.

Again, this is our innate biology and response to stress working for our benefit. This is why modern women have a tendency to talk about their problems and share in order to feel safe and reach resolution.

Have you noticed the juxtaposition of how males and females deal with stress? They are opposite, and in today's world can become a source of conflict or misunderstanding between partners.

I talk about this now in order to lay the foundation for understanding and awareness of how you both communicate. It was so easy to make love and now you are joyfully pregnant, but you have to make some decisions about how and where and with whom you want to give birth. While you are exploring your birth journey choices, keep in mind the innate difference in communication styles between you and your partner.

Meanwhile, back at the ancestral village, our Grandmother of Grandmother of Grandmothers is fully pregnant and has just completed her blessing way rite of passage to motherhood. The council of Grandmothers is in charge of the ceremony and preparing for the eventual birth. The mothers who have given birth before are helping, for they know that someday they, too, will become Grandmothers and join the council of elders.

Everything in the village is always planned in community with Gaia: Mother Earth, Pachamama, and the Giver of Life to all humanity. Many activities are planned around the seasons. Birth journeys are no different.

As women, we cycle with the moon and are more likely to give birth when the moon is at its fullest. This is still a warning for labor units in today's modern life. With the full moon, it is easier to see at night, a time when most women tend to deliver. This is still true even today, especially in the hot months of summer. At the beginning of your Grandmother's labor, the village women gather with her by the water's edge.

Ancient Birth Ritual

Now as you envision this birth scene, look very closely at your young "Grandmother's" face. You are in for a surprise – she looks just like you! And you may have a keen sense that you were her in a past life, long ago when life was simple and in harmony with nature. Let your mind's eye see yourself as her during the ancient birth ritual. You will now experience the beauty of an ancient birth ritual.

*****

All the women know that a lagoon or gentle pond's shallow waters is always the best place to labor and give birth. While in the water, you remember feeling weightless, and you could easily lean on your birth sisters in attendance during the rushes of energy going through your body. In between the rushes, you would talk with your sisters, move your hips back and forth, and maybe even do belly dance movements to help the time go by more joyfully and with ease.

Maybe all of you would chant and sing songs of strength and awareness of new life entering the world. Then there were quiet times when all the women would focus lovingly and peacefully on your needs while they encouraged you and reminded you to breathe. Take notice of the trees and feel the breeze on your face and through your hair.

Sometimes, you would get out of the water and go to the birth tree. This is where the midwives had hung a rope or cloth that you could easily grab during some intense rushes to let your lower body move freely while you wiggled your hips from side to side without having to fully stand on your feet.

You were free to eat and drink water and herbal teas that were made available to you. You had no worries, for you had helped other women go through the same process and now it was your turn to be the goddess of birth.

Now you start to feel pressure low in your pelvis during the rushes of energy traveling downward in your body toward Gaia. Instinctively you know it's time to let the water support your body once again with the help of your sister's the midwives, women being with woman (the meaning of "midwife") at your side.

With every rush of your contracting uterus, you bear down and naturally reach between your legs to support your perineum. You start to feel the top of your baby's head, which is confirmed by one of the midwives. You continue to gently push until the head is born and then the shoulders follow; you reach down and pull the rest of your baby to your bare chest.

With great joy, all of you greet your new baby, who is healthily crying and moving its outstretched arms and little fingers towards your face. Your midwives guide you out of the water so you can lie on a blanket near the birth tree. While they cover and dry both you and the baby, your baby instinctively finds your breast and starts to nurse.

The main midwife is monitoring how both of you are doing and checks for a pulse in the cord connecting the baby to the undelivered placenta. She finds that the pulse has stopped and your baby is happily breastfeeding, so she ties off the umbilical cord and cuts the baby free.

Shortly thereafter, you start to feel another rush of contractions and pressure in your bottom. One quick strong push and out comes your placenta. The midwives save the placenta, because they will preserve it with salt and let it dehydrate, and then grind it down to a powder that you will later ingest to help keep your postpartum hormones in balance. You can still find women who know how to do this today.

This is how we were made to give birth, and it's still how we're made to give birth today in the 21st century. Yet we are slowly losing our way. Somehow, we need to go back to the way our bodies know to give birth.

Your Birth Akashic Records

Surprisingly, this birth story from long ago seems so familiar, doesn't it? That's because it is deep in your Akashic Records. You may be asking, what are Akashic Records? Well let's say you are open to the possibility of reincarnation. So, with that in mind, I will briefly give you a surface explanation.

"Akash" is a word derived from the Sanskrit word *Akasha*, which has different meanings depending on the philosophy you follow. The basic meaning of the word Akash is the sky, space, and ether in an elemental and metaphysical sense, representing our own personal mystical knowledge that we carry encoded in our genes and in the non-physical plane of existence.

Therefore, our human Akashic Records are within us in our DNA and outside of us in Gaia (Earth). Both our DNA and Gaia hold the records of our many lives on this earth, and those can be retrieved by going within and tapping into the infinite wisdom of our higher self. The part of you that is always connected to God, the Universe, and Spirit is your higher self. This is also the multi-dimensional plane that you can access when you meditate.

You can learn more about these concepts from the books *The Gaia Effect* and *The Human Akash* by Kyron and Monika Muranyi. Here is an excerpt from the latter book that will better explain the concepts.

"When you pass through the 'wind of birth' and take your first breath, your unique life expression begins. The Akash is an energy that comes in with you. The term 'Akashic Record' is a record of the Akash. The Akash can be defined as an energy that represents 'all that is.' Your Akashic Record is therefore a record of everything you have ever been and more. The concept of the Akash also represents the potentials of everything that can be, things that are potentially unrealized."

~ *THE HUMAN AKASH*

BY KRYON AND MONIKA MURANYI.

In short, I have found that it's important for me and my clients to not underestimate the impact of our past lives, especially if they come up organically as part of the healing process. We are part of the collective consciousness of the planet. We are one, which makes it possible to have remembrance of your own Grandmother of Grandmothers in a village long ago, and of her birth experience. It may have been as pristine as the one described, or it may have been the opposite. Either way, with these techniques my clients can tap into their collective consciousness and access resources for healing events of their current life.

My clients use those memories to heal the negative emotions that are still connected to the past. It is possible to reach back into their own Akashic Records and heal any previous birth struggles or retrieve birth triumphs. This is part of the healing process I guide my clients through. I have found this to be very powerful and have seen it create a change in the energetic potential of my clients' lives and empowered birth journeys.

Become your own ancestor! This is a wonderful process to getting the birth of your dreams. Write a love letter to your future self-describing all the details of the dream birth that your future self will experience. Watch your wording and do not include any "don't do this" and "don't do that" language. I will explain later why this is so important.

*****

Love Letter Exercise

Give yourself a moment to write this letter to your future self and make it all about love, peace, and kindness as you describe your future birth journey. Date your letter and put it in an envelope for safekeeping, or include it in your journaling. Keep track of where you put it, because we will be referring to it at the end of the book.

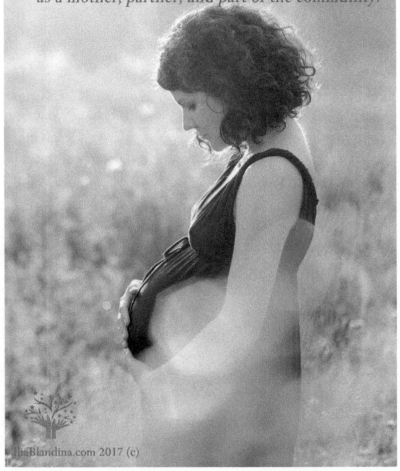

The birth process is incredibly important to a woman.
It's an amazing and beautiful time,
and a life-altering opportunity
that becomes a defining moment
in your life and for who you become
as a mother, partner, and part of the community.

CHAPTER 2

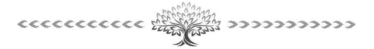

Sacred Birth

"So many gods, so many creeds,
So many paths that wind and wind,
While just the art of being kind,
Is all this sad world needs.
~ ELLA WHEELER WILCOX

Connecting to Your Divine Biology

n pregnancy, you have the unique opportunity of creating a new life that will help humanity. You not only experience the birth of your baby, but you also can potentiate the rebirth of yourself. It is a mystical and sacred time in your life that may only happen once, twice, three, or four times – however many babies you are planning for, or maybe you follow the philosophy of letting God give you as many as is spiritually determined. Either way, it is still a finite number of opportunities to truly commune with the mysteries of the Divine.

Just imagine for a moment: out of all the two million immature eggs you were born with, 75% have died off by the time you reach puberty. It will take 1000 of the remaining 500,000 to begin to mature each month in order to create that one egg that gets released from your ovary – and its size is that of the period at the end of this sentence. As your egg travels from your ovary into your fallopian tube, it floats into and through your uterus, available for fertilization for only 24 hours.

If the timing is just right, at some point during its floating journey through your fallopian tube, your mature egg will be greeted by 100 million sperm, all of which will poke and prod the membrane of the egg hoping to be The One that is let in.

Yes, the egg will do the choosing. Once the one sperm is chosen, the father's DNA is extracted and joins with your DNA. Then rapid cell division begins while the egg becomes a zygote on the rest of its float down into the uterine cavity. This journey and miracle of transformation lasts for seven days after fertilization. It is like a microscopic space voyage.

Eventually, the zygote will land on the soft surface of your uterine lining, a nutrient-dense area where it will attach to your very own blood supply. Voilá! During the next 11 weeks, the zygote will need to be supported by the hormones released from your ovaries until the placenta has developed and matured enough to take over the hormone production.

The miracle continues: after implantation, the zygote becomes an embryo, then, at 12 weeks' gestational age, a fetus. Maybe somewhere around eight weeks' gestational age you might have noticed you were late with your cycle and decided to get a pregnancy test. We all know how this goes, but have you really considered how much occurred between ovulation to conception to implantation and then to "Oh, I'm pregnant!"? It truly is a miracle and mystical experience that we are continuing to study and be amazed by.

Why am I getting into this whole human biology 101? Just as a point of reference to say how magical life is. The beginning is so silent and unseen, yet from this beginning starts the sacred foundation of the human family. Our pregnancy and birth journey is the start of all that is sacred on the Earth. We must guard and reclaim the empowered births of our families.

Birth as Empowerment for Women

The birth process is incredibly important to a woman. It's an amazing and beautiful time, and a life-altering opportunity that becomes a defining moment in your life and for who you become as a mother, partner, and part of the community.

Your birth journey will transform you, like it or not. For as long as you live, you will remember how you felt during your births. Birth can be incredible, empowering, and beautiful; or it can leave you feeling disempowered, traumatized, and scarred (literally and figuratively).

For many, it is a rite of passage. Nothing compares to the privilege of giving birth and the responsibility of it all. You are literally transported into another realm. For as much as you arrange to be surrounded by people who will support and keep your journey safe, it still is an internal quest of courage and endurance, a sacred journey into motherhood, and a shamanic teaching for your baby. All that you experience will be imprinted in your baby's experience.

You go deep into yourself when you are in labor and you discover things about yourself that you may not have known before. You even learn things on birth two, three, or four that will impact your life forever and make you a stronger, more courageous, and more resilient person.

The birth process helps you to learn how your body works, and this is very important in our journey as mothers. Birth is best approached from a point of view of not wanting to minimize the experience. Instead prepare yourself to embrace the whole experience and all the mystery, suspense, and challenges.

Along the way, what I have learned from my clients is that their own attitude and what they pay attention to during labor actually affects the course of their labor. This is why it is good practice to create a sacred space for labor to occur. The best space you can control is your home and the next best is a birth center, but the least controllable environment is the hospital. Besides creating a sacred space outside of your body, it is just as important to create a sacred space inside your body.

Communication with Your Baby

The most effective way to create your internal sacred space is to learn how to control your innermost thoughts and emotions. I teach my clients to move into a more peaceful state of mind throughout their pregnancy.

What's most important is that you engage in some form of daily meditation and ritual that will help you practice mindfulness. By being your own sacred witness, you allow any negative emotions to be released so that you can provide your baby inside your womb with a peaceful environment.

Yes, your emotional environment can affect the baby. This idea is supported by the latest evidence from psychology and biology. The most important teaching we do with our babies is done before birth, during pregnancy.

During this special time, we as mothers become the shamans to our unborn children. The health and wellbeing of our baby's life is crucially affected by the nine months they spend in the womb. Our babies learn about the outside world before they are born. What we experience while pregnant is taught to our babies in various ways.

First, our babies learn the sound of our voices, starting at around four months' gestation. Although muted and muffled while traveling from the outside in through your womb, your voice reverberates through your body very readily to reach your baby.

Your voice and heart beat is what your baby hears the most. Your baby is with you all the time, therefore, after birth, your baby recognizes your voice and prefers to listen to you above all others.

Researchers tested this by rigging up two rubber nipples. If the baby sucked on one, it would hear a recording of its mom's voice through headphones. If it sucked on the other nipple, the baby would hear the voice of a female stranger. Babies quickly showed they preferred their mom's voice!

Another study showed that after women repeatedly read a section of Dr. Seuss's *The Cat in the Hat* aloud while they were pregnant, their newborns would recognize that passage when they heard it outside the womb by slowing down their sucking, which is something they commonly do when something interests them. Babies have also been known to recognize TV show theme songs if their mother watched the show every day while pregnant.

Babies are also learning the family's native language. A study published by Dr. Kathleen Wermke of the University of Wurzbirg, Germany and colleagues looked at the patterns of baby cries in the first five days of life and reported it in the journal *Current Biology*. The researchers noticed French baby cries tended to start low and end in a raised pitch, while German baby cries tended to start high and end low in pitch.

These attributes at birth help the baby's survival by promoting the ability to respond to the voice of the person who will most likely be the main caregiver, mom. Not only do the babies learn their native language, but they also learn the tastes and flavors of their native foods. These flavors find their way into the amniotic fluid, which the baby is always drinking while in the womb.

One study looked at two groups of mothers. One group drank carrot juice a lot during pregnancy, and the other only water. At six months old, the babies whose mom drank carrot juice preferred carrot-flavored cereal, while the other babies whose mom drank water did not prefer the carrot cereal.

A similar study was done with the flavor of anise, and the same results occurred. The babies exposed to anise while in the womb liked its flavor after birth on their first day of life while the other babies hated the flavor.

How Babies Learn to Survive

There are even bigger lessons babies learn. One large study of the effects of extreme malnutrition on 40,000 pregnant mothers who had to endure a year of food rations in Holland during World War II found that decades later, the babies who reached adulthood were more prone to obesity, diabetes, and heart disease.

When food is scarce in the womb, fetuses adapt by diverting nutrients to the brain and away from other organs like the heart and pancreas, and that means they are more susceptible to disease. While enduring the harsh environment produced by their mothers' food deprivation, the fetuses adjusted their body chemistry to hang onto every calorie.

Another study followed 1700 pregnant women who witnessed the 9/11 terror attack on the World Trade Center firsthand. The women, who developed posttraumatic stress syndrome (PTSD) while pregnant, had babies that tested positive for a biological marker of PTSD susceptibility at just one year of age. It's as if the moms who witnessed 9/11 were giving their unborn babies a heads-up that it may not be safe out here, so you need the tools to be hyper-vigilant.

The point here is not to have you walk away with feelings of guilt and fear. My intention, instead, is to make you aware that from the very beginning; your baby is listening to you and interacting with your hormonal environment. So, it is a very important practice to keep your environment sacred and as serene as possible. Don't let yourself stew in stress and negative emotions. Remember your emotional and hormonal soup is also being given to your baby.

Sacred Bonding Before Birth

Developing a sacred bond with your baby during pregnancy will allow you to use this bond right from the start of labor by imagining a joint effort with your baby. In essence, you can teach your baby to be your partner during birth.

I always tell my clients to start a bedtime ritual. Lie on your side and practice visualizing the birth of your baby. Imagine a quick and painless birth with your baby helping you during labor. Of course, if you are concerned that you may trigger preterm labor you can state it like this: "I see myself having a quick and easy birth within two days of my due date of [insert date here]."

You may say things out loud while you are in labor to your baby like: Hurry and come out; I can't wait to meet you; I want to see you; and let's work together so you can finally meet your new family. Tap on your meridian points, which I'll explain in Chapter 7, to infuse these positive thoughts into your body.

When you are not yet full term, you can still meditate on how your baby might look and what position they are in, and tell your baby you are looking forward to seeing them in [fill in your delivery month]. Use belly butters and before you fall asleep, rub your belly and talk to your baby while you tap on your meridian points. All these thoughts and practices help form a deep, sacred connection with your baby before birth, one that will help with the pain and work of labor.

This sacred connection is different than the one you have with your partner. Practicing holding the image of your loving baby as a labor partner creates the feeling of a joint effort, sacred connection, and purpose. After all, you created this partnership before you were both born. In other words, the soul of your baby and your soul made an agreement to be mother and child before either of you arrived here on earth.

Part of the process I teach my clients is to develop a relationship with the incoming soul long before birth, and I have found this to ease the transition of the baby into this world.

Parenting is one of the most profound spiritual roles available to us and it can begin before the birth. Creating a sacred birth environment combines the intense physical experience of pregnancy and your empowered birth journey with the spiritual experience of welcoming a soul into the body and attuning your hearts together.

I'll tell you a lot more about this later in this book, but for now, here's a brief overview of how you might create that sacred birth environment for you and your baby.

At the start of labor, you may begin by opening sacred space. You can practice opening sacred space before labor, when you do mindfulness meditation or any of the tapping sequences I'll explain in Chapter 8. You can open sacred space by any means that you are comfortable with. One of my favorite ways is to use a prayer that invites the energy of the four directions. I've included this as part of my downloadable VBAC Tool Kit, if you would like to use it.

After opening your personal sacred space, you can use sage or palo santo to smudge all who participate in your birth. You can also designate special candles that have been blessed with your birth intentions and light them while you are in labor. Now depending on the location, you have picked for your birth, you may not be able to have a burning flame, but even if you plan a hospital birth, the first part of your labor should be at home. The goal is always to stay at home as long as possible. The explanation in Chapter 5 will help you to see why this is so important.

Things to consider during labor to ease the sensation of your rushes and surges (contractions) is to have someone else be your time keeper. Your primary job is to stay as peaceful as possible during your journey. *"A watched pot does not boil"* and this holds true with labor as well. So, plan to keep your eyes off the clock, instead you can look at one of the many images in the VBAC Tool Kit or use your own favorite image as a focal point.

Consider having some easy songs to sing, it helps to keep your jaw relaxed and that helps your cervix to open. Have a tub full of warm water or use your hot tub at lower temperatures (like a warm bath). A warm bath is very relaxing in labor and has been shown to alter the perception of pain.

Remember to walk, eat when hungry and drink plenty of water and juices for energy. Keep your surroundings quiet and don't allow people to pop in and out. Have your partner rub your back if it makes you feel better. This is especially important if you tend to feel your rushes and surges in your low back. I will be addressing what to do if you think you are having back labor in Chapter 6.

You can also create or incorporate any ceremonies or prayers from your personal spiritual belief system. The main goal is to create a memorable and positive emotional atmosphere of love and support.

After the baby is born and all is settled if you have opened sacred space, remember to close it by reciting the same prayer and adding, "You may go and thank you for being with us." Creating ritual with your birth journey helps you to learn life lessons that will impact the relationship of the whole family.

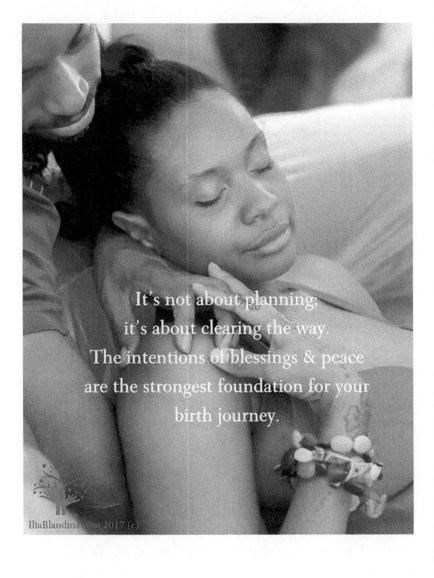

It's not about planning;
it's about clearing the way.
The intentions of blessings & peace
are the strongest foundation for your
birth journey.

IliaBlandina Bowen 2017 (c)

CHAPTER 3

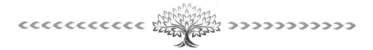

Creating the
Perfect Birth Plan

*"When we speak, we are afraid our words will not be heard
or welcomed. But when we are silent, we are still afraid. So,
it is better to speak."*

~ AUDRE LORDE

Law of Attraction and Birth Plans

There is nothing like the courage of putting your feelings into
words. I was once trapped into thinking that I had to conform
to the conventional rules of how to give birth after a C-section
because I was a midwife in the hospital system. I then realized it was
time to spread my wings and use my power through words.

As a midwife, I have helped many women cope with all the rules of
birth in a hospital setting, but as a client, I sought to give birth either

at home or a birth center, including having my VBAC at home. I feel it is time to pass on the knowledge and understanding of the power of our words.

Through my own births and the many women, I helped, I came to understand how the words we use are very powerful and can affect our own birth outcomes. This realization made me feel like it was time to spread our wings by teaching how the power of the words we use when preparing for birth can create a new birth outcome reality. This is done through The Law of Attraction and the power of intention.

The Law of Attraction as it relates to achieving an empowered birth journey is a very powerful tool. First you must clearly understand what the Law of Attraction is. It is a maxim that means "like attracts like," which means that focusing on positive or negative thoughts brings positive or negative experiences into your birth journey.

The Law of Attraction has its basis in quantum physics, a science studied by many, including physicist Sir Roger Penrose and Stuart Hameroff, MD, Director of Consciousness Studies at the University of Arizona. Our brain fires neurons that produce thoughts in response to our environment. Those thoughts, in turn, influence that environment.

Thoughts and words have been found to have a unique wave form pattern, which means they have their own unique frequency and energy signature. Because we are conscious beings, when we use our thoughts and words with an intention for a specific outcome, we can match the frequency of the reality we want and attract that reality to us. This happens subconsciously or consciously, so the aim is to become conscious of our thoughts in order to attract the empowered birth we desire.

At the end of this chapter you will see a list of Do's and Don'ts. It's not an exhaustive list, but it will effectively illustrate how the Law of Attraction does not differentiate between positive or negative requests. When you understand that the Law of Attraction doesn't distinguish between "hard" and "not hard," you can clearly see why birth plans can be jinxed from the start.

Please don't misunderstand me. Yes, let your needs be known – but watch the language you use to request what you want. Birth plans that focus on what we *don't* want are birth plans many labor nurses, including hospital midwives, do not like reading because they are aware that by stating what you don't want, is basically tell the universe that you do want it. Many times, these "I don't want this or that" birth plans are met by nervous laughter from the staff on labor and delivery units and instead become a warning of how your labor may not go as planned.

So, the key is to stay away from fear-based requests such as "I don't want [xyz]." Instead, state your needs positively: "If safety allows, [xyz] is what I want to see happen during my birth journey." Let your needs and desires be known, but construct the language in a positive, empowering, and flexible way. Focus on your needs instead of trying to micro-manage the details of medical care.

You don't have control over all the possible outcomes, and that should not be your focus anyway. You *do* have the right to complete informed consent (or informed refusal), so that you can move toward forming the vision of your empowered VBAC. Do your homework ahead of time and pick practitioners and a birth setting that you completely trust and who will truly listen to your requests and needs.

*****

I always teach my clients my motto when it comes to birth plans: *It's not about planning; it's about clearing the way.*

Your Empowered Birth Journey

First and foremost, enter into your birth journey by realizing you are not alone. Even if by some strange turn of events you are physically alone (the most common time is when your birth partner has to take a break and suddenly the contraction from hell arrives), always know that God, Angels, and your ancestors are there with you in Spirit.

I teach my clients to control how they respond and feel about all the horror stories they may have heard from friends or relatives. By being able to control their negative emotions, my clients are able to access the knowledge of those ancestors who came before them.

On our planet, we forget the power of Gaia herself, we forget how so many women came before us and gave birth naturally. It was a rite of passage, not a crisis. We have the power of pure intention and creation though our ability to own our birth journey.

Think of your birth plan as a path of intentions instead of a directive. The plan should begin with this statement: *I intend my empowered birth journey to be safe and peaceful. With this in mind and if safety allows, the following list is what I want to see happen during my birth journey.* Intention means getting clear about what you want. There is no room for what you don't want. Forget about what you don't want.

Here is the big secret: practitioners don't want what you don't want – and by "what you don't want," I mean a bad outcome. So, there is no need to bring it up. That's how the best-laid plans get jinxed. Everyone involved wants that quintessential peaceful, powerful, and loving birth. Believe it or not, we are all starting on the same page. Let's stay there by focusing on your intention for your birth journey.

Intention and Your Birth Journey

What gets in the way of formulating and holding our birth journey intentions is that our minds start overanalyzing under the influence of rising stress hormones. We get stuck in what we don't want to happen, and then surprise, it happens anyway. You start to think, I want this but I want it under these conditions, I don't want to lose that and it can't affect this and if this occurs then this is going to happen, and on and on it goes.

If you focus on the limitations of planning your birth instead of the freedom you want, you lose sight of the end goal. Trust me: ultimately, you will not be able to control everything. The Universe, God, and Spirit do not work like that. What you can control is the image you hold in your mind of the intention of your birth journey.

Intention is when you contemplate, "What would it be like to have a peaceful and loving birth?" The moment you ask that open-ended question, your frontal lobe, which is 40% of your brain and its creative center, starts to kick into gear. Your brain starts to work on the possibility and your creative center turns on and looks over all the different stored memories, whether you are conscious of them or not.

These different networks of neurons are stored in your brain based on what you have learned intellectually or experienced in the past: "I know what it's like to be in labor and no matter how well I prepared myself, I still got a C-section." "I know what it is like to have a vaginal exam and I hate it." "I don't like people to see me naked."

Your brain starts to call up all these different memory networks and it seamlessly puts them together to create a new idea, a new vision. *"And when you put all those networks together and they fire in tandem, you will get a clear picture in your mind. And that clear picture is called intention."* ~ Dr. Joe Dispenza.

Herein lies the problem. The more negative conditions or negative specifics you have about your birth experience, the more you will attract the negative picture. This is when you have to take note of the negative emotions and events that are coming up about your previous birth experiences.

I help my clients do this by guiding them to verbalize their specific fears and by teaching them tapping techniques called Emotional

Freedom Techniques (EFT). I will explain how these techniques work in Chapter 7.

Clearing Negative Emotions

Setting a clear intention is to overcome any negative emotional ties you have in your past that block you from developing a clear picture of your future. After clearing your negative emotional triggers, you are ready to create your personal Birth Journey Intention list. All the elements of your list will become elements to add to the vision of your birth.

The picture in your mind could be easily represented by one image or even one word. For my clients, I created the program and imagery of a "Childbirth With Grace" that looks like this:

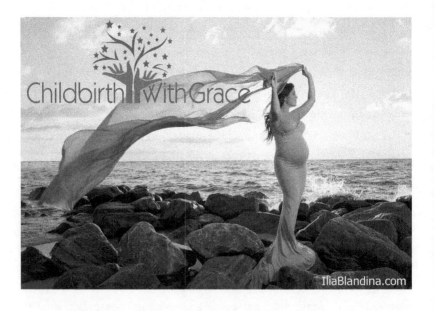

After you formulate your Birth Journey Intention list, start to use the list while you are meditating and tapping. Make a recording of your intentions and play them with soft music in the background. This will help you see the birth of your dreams. In essence, you can have several conditions that make up your intention, but the intention itself is typically a symbol or image that represents all of your conditions.

In that moment when you can see the birth of your dreams and you have a picture of it in your mind, you can then start to live your dream birth. After practicing these techniques, you start to take the dream birth and turn it into a motion picture. Now you are *in* that imaginary birth.

When your dream birth journey starts to take form, it also transcends time; you will start to experience it and all the things you are going to do. This process allows you to live in that future, and that's important, because your brain does not know the difference between the actual events taking place in your life and the imagined birth in your mind. This is called mental rehearsal. In the practice of doing this during your meditations and tapping, you are literally rewiring yourself to the future that contains your quintessential birth experience.

Imprinting Positive Emotions

Now you need to imagine the emotions that come with your empowered birth experience. This will make the intentions come alive. Your body is your unconscious mind and when you combine vision with emotion your body will not know the difference between an experience in your life that creates an emotion and an emotion that you created by just visualizing it.

This practice will help your body, as it reflects your unconscious mind, to live in the future of your dream birth while in the present moment and you will epigenetically change your body (an epigenetic change is anything that influences an organism above a DNA level) to be able to adapt in preparation for the birth you are imagining.

Here is another secret: You have to want this birth to happen. What I mean is, there is no room for fear or doubt. You can't wait for the dream birth to physically happen, you have to feel it happening in your mind, you have to see it happen, you have to practice living it.

You can't wait to feel empowered about your birth; you have to feel empowered now in the present moment. Most women wait for something outside of them to change how they feel about birth, but this is an outdated, cause-and-effect model of reality. What I am talking about here is the quantum model of reality, which means that you will need to change how you think about birth before the experience occurs in order for your dream birth to find you.

The best emotion you can cultivate to be included in your birth experience is love. So, what you will need to do is bring love, kindness, and peace with you so that in turn, you will receive it back during your birth.

If you only bring fear and doubt, then that very thing you don't want will be mirrored back at you. Yes, fear and doubt may lead to another C-section. During the labor process your senses are heightened and so are your birth attendants. If you don't have resolution regarding your fear and doubts, they can seep into the birth environment from either you or your practitioner. When this happens, you can get into a pattern of mirroring back to each other the very same fear and doubt that both of you are projecting. This scenario feeds into the Fear-Tension-Pain cycle that prohibits labor from progressing.

"... so, if your personality creates your personal reality and your personality is made up of how you think and how you act and how you feel; the present personality who [is reading this book] has created the present personal reality called their life. So, if they wanted to create a new personal reality in their life, they would have to start thinking about what they are thinking about and changing. Starting to become conscious of their unconscious habits and behaviors and modify them."

~ DR. JOE DISPENZA

EXCERPT OF YOUTUBE VIDEO, DR. JOE DISPENZA *DEFINING INTENTION*

The key is you have to look at the emotions you have memorized and that are keeping you anchored to your past birth experiences and you have to decide whether they are serving you and whether they fit into your future birth journey.

Think back to your first birth. If you had a plan, did your birth go accordingly? If not, try to make connections between the personality you had then and the birth you had. See how it matches up? So, with this birth, let's identify how you would have to change to get the birth you want. The overall goal is to re-identify with your future birth journey, instead of bringing the past or present with you. This requires a tremendous amount of awareness.

"Awareness means then to have to stay conscious and pay attention to who you are being all the time and you can't let any thoughts slip by your awareness that's going to cause you to return back to the old self. You can't begin to react emotionally to people and things in your life that cause you to feel like the old self. You can't talk and complain and blame and make excuses or go back to old habits and expect your future to show up. You have to maintain that state for a period of time so that your body catches up, because the body and brain live in the past. It takes a certain amount of repetition and a certain amount of consciousness, a certain amount of will to finally arrive there and I am happy to say that it is possible."

~ DR. JOE DISPENZA

BREAKING THE HABIT OF BEING YOURSELF

Physical and Practical Magic for Your Birth Journey

One way to generate positive and uplifting emotions is by listening to music. Before labor is a good time to gather up music that evokes empowering emotions for your birth experience. For example, as I write this chapter, I am listening to "Earth" by Hans Zimmer, from the music of the motion picture *Gladiator*. Sounds counter-intuitive, maybe, but I've always seen myself as a warrior of birth, so it resonates with my personal vision of my own births. I invite you to start exploring your personal vision and voice of your birth journey.

And now for some physical and practical advice: Things you should include in your personal birth kit and why.

Watch funny movies or shows

Laughter will release endorphins, hormones equivalent to morphine. Every time you laugh during labor, you are giving yourself a dose of natural pain relief!

By the same token, avoid horror or thriller movies and TV shows. Scary movies will trigger your stress hormones of fight, flight, or freeze, which is the release of adrenaline, and those hormones cause the muscle of your uterus to soften and stop contracting. Unless you want to stop your labor, do not watch any thrillers or scary stuff.

Make a rice bag and put your favorite aromatherapy blend in it

Check out the VBAC Tool Kit, which includes directions on how to make an aromatherapy rice bag for labor. I used this personally during my VBAC home birth and it was equivalent to having an epidural. The pain was numbed away!

Learn some easy songs or chants you can vocalize during birth

When you keep your throat open, this also allows your cervix to soften and open. You can Google "goddess chants" and find many ancient verses. The one below is very old and the author is unknown. It was featured in the documentary *Birth Story.*

Open
I am feeling very open
Like a flower in the morn
Let my petals open
Let my child be born

EFT can also be used to control cravings during pregnancy

This in turn will help control your overall weight gain and therefore the size of your baby; a very important tip especially if your C-section was done because you were told your baby was too big to deliver vaginally.

The size of your baby is one of the most common reasons why elective C-sections are performed. It's like a pre-emptive strike to try to avoid shoulder dystocia (the baby's shoulders getting stuck under the pubic bone).

Be very careful about how you write your birth plan

Now it's time to look at the "Dos & Don'ts" list. Read them out loud as they are listed. Notice when you read them out loud that without interjecting the "I do want" or "I don't want" words in front of the items in both lists, it sounds like you want all of it to happen. This is precisely how Universe or Spirit hears your requests. Whether you "do" want it or you "don't" want it, you will get it.

Forget about what you "don't" want, concentrate, visualize and imagine what you "do" want. When my clients find this hard to do, it is because they are still caught up in the negative emotions of the past, I coach them to help release those negative emotions before they go into labor.

Do's:

- Think of birth as a sacred family event
- Believe in your intuition and your innate ability to give birth
- Connect with your higher self; she always knows what to do
- Connect with empowering women
- Get rid of negative birth thinkers; they are not invited
- Believe there is a special energy surrounding birth
- Laugh, Sing, Dance, Walk, Soak in a warm tub
- Change your language about birth; a contraction can be called a "rush" or "wave"
- Increase physical relaxation
- Breath slowly and stay calm
- Use aromatherapy and rice bags
- Drink red raspberry tea with honey
- Use mantras and chants
- Increase your love hormones (oxytocin)
- Keep the room calm; surround yourself with advocates for a calm environment (sort of like a hall monitor)
- Enjoy your birth experience

Don'ts:

- Be afraid of birth
- Let yourself be talked into a c-section
- Think birth is gross
- Think doctors know everything about natural birth (unless they use to be a nurse or midwife)
- Listen to scary birth stories
- Underestimate the presence of compassionate people
- Increase your stress hormones (cortisol)
- Regret your past experiences and revisit them often
- Equate pain with birth
- Panic and be alone
- Stay with people you don't trust
- Make rigid birth plans
- Let people scare you out of what you want
- Assume that repeat c-sections are safer
- Assume that induction of labor is safer than waiting for labor to start on its own

Read the above items in both lists out loud and you will be very surprised how it will come across that you are asking for both the positive and negative to happen. That is how the Law of Attraction can jinx your birth plan. Remember, *"It's not about planning; it's about clearing the way."*

The power of belief in yourself is your greatest gift.
Don't let anyone take that from you.
Follow your instincts.

CHAPTER 4

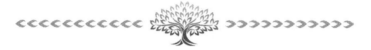

The Power of Belief

"The most common way people give up their power is by thinking they don't have any."
~ ALICE WALKER

The Shadow Birth Journey

You can live your dreams, or you can live your fears. Let me ask you this: what are you afraid of when you dare to see yourself giving birth vaginally? This is the belief you have to explore in order to have emotional freedom in your birth journey of having a VBAC.

The key is that in order to change your belief, you have to identify the fears that feed it. Don't worry; identifying your fears won't make them come true. Instead, you will shed light on them and be able to resolve the core belief of your fears' foundation. This will change your belief and overcome your fears; this is your true power.

Shortly after creating a Facebook page for this book, I received a message from a friend: "Yikes. My friend did a VBAC and her uterus exploded during labor. Baby now has brain damage." With this in mind, I decided to tackle this most common fear when it comes to choosing whether to proceed with a trial of labor after cesarean.

My response to the message was: "I'm so sorry. There are many reasons that may have happened for your friend. But the risk of that outcome is very low. There is even a risk of uterine rupture during normal vaginal birth with no history of a previous cesarean. Risk is difficult to predict."

You can have very low odds, perhaps a one in a million chance, but if you are that one, then it becomes a 100% chance for you. Overall, it is impossible to eliminate all risk from life or birth, therefore every choice has its risks and benefits. All we can do as women is to choose the risk that intuitively feels right for us. We need to emotionally reconcile that there are no risk-free choices.

The purpose and intention of this book is to bring awareness to how women can let go of negative, fear-based thinking and negative emotions so that they are better able to make the decisions that feel right for them.

Making decisions in a state of fear-based thinking limits your perspective and thereby limits your choices. There are many ways of presenting risks, and some may be biased either for or against a VBAC and the risk of uterine rupture. The numbers can be presented from both points of view.

Here's an example. If we look at the overall risk of uterine rupture after having had a single previous C-section (without accounting for specific factors like the use of Pitocin or any type of uterine scar or closure technique), the numbers can be presented in different ways such as:

- 50 out of 10,000 will have a uterine rupture

- 9950 out of 10,000 will not have a uterine rupture
- One in 200 will have a uterine rupture
- 199 out of 200 will not have a uterine rupture
- Overall percent chance of a uterine rupture is 0.5%
- Overall percent chance of not having a uterine rupture is 99.5%

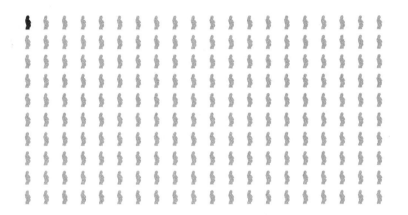

It basically comes down to which version of the numbers feel right for you. *"Is the cup half empty or half full?"* Actually, the odds are in favor of the cup being more than half full. Personally, I was willing to take the risk that I would be in the 99.5% group when I made my decision to have a VBAC at home. Mind you, I knew exactly what my risks were, having been a certified nurse midwife for many years, including having done many C-sections on clients as the first-assist surgeon.

Placebo vs. Nocebo

Let's talk about the placebo versus the nocebo affect. First the definitions:

- A placebo is a harmless pill, medicine, or procedure prescribed more for the psychological benefit to the patient than for any physiological effect. Placebos are usually used as a control in testing new drugs. A placebo can also be defined as a measure designed to calm or please someone. In Latin it means, "I shall please."
- A nocebo is a detrimental effect on health produced by psychological or psychosomatic factors such as negative expectations of treatment or prognosis. In Latin it means, "I shall cause harm."

It's important to know these concepts and to understand their potential influence on your own beliefs. Henry Ford's famous quote, *"Whether you think you can or you think you can't, you're right,"* holds very true during the birth process.

Here is the caveat: you have to establish your personal belief in yourself far in advance of labor or else you risk that someone else will plant the seed of doubt in your ability to birth vaginally.

In clinical trials, the placebo effect is noted when patients experience the healing effect of a new drug or surgery even though they were getting a fake treatment. The placebo effect is real and works anywhere from 18 to 80% of the time!

It's not in your head, either. Studies have found that placebos have actually dilated bronchi, healed ulcers, eliminated warts, lowered blood pressure, and even grown hair on the heads of balding men who think they are using Rogaine!

New drugs are approved to go to market by performing at least 1% better than the placebo, and the placebo just has to work 30% of the time. Isn't that interesting? In other words, practitioners and the FDA have no problem prescribing or releasing to market a medication that may fail *69% of the time*. This is an oversimplification, but you get what I am saying. All you have to do for a drug to work is BELIEVE.

Now let's talk about the shadow side of the placebo "I shall please" effect. Its dark underbelly side is the nocebo "I shall cause harm" effect. The same mind-body connection that can make you successful at a VBAC can also make you fail a trial of labor.

When patients in many double-blind clinical trials are warned about side effects they may experience if they are given the experimental drug, about 25% experience the most severe side effects, even if they are given the sugar pill.

The powerful finding is that nocebo effects are not random; they tend to match the warnings given to the test subjects before treatment. In one study, patients who were given saline but believed they were given chemotherapy actually vomited and lost their hair! This should be a light bulb moment for you. It certainly was for me!

I saw the placebo and nocebo effects again and again in my practice as a midwife. As a practitioner, I knew the power of my ability to suggest a certain outcome. I would only advise my clients in a positive way, unless there was an emergency. Meanwhile, I had no power over what my consulting physician would say when I called them to evaluate my clients.

When those physicians would tell my clients that they did not believe my clients could have a vaginal birth, but that they would give them a couple of hours to see if the labor would progress? Well, most of the time, it became a self-fulfilling prophecy. Doctors do not intentionally mean to cause harm; they just think they are giving you a warning ahead of time, so that you won't be disappointed when C-section time comes.

How strong is the placebo versus the nocebo effect? Interestingly, studies that look at the expectation of diminishing pain (the placebo effect) usually show a very strong placebo effect at onset, but those positive effects diminish fairly rapidly, probably because the relationship between the placebo intervention and the decreased pain experience is no longer being reinforced.

In contrast, when studies look at the nocebo effect, where subjects are told the intervention will cause them pain even though it really isn't a painful intervention, not only do people feel pain, but the increased pain to the nocebo intervention did not diminish over time, unlike the placebo effect that did diminish over time.

These studies were looking at interventions that either alleviated pain or caused pain. So the finding that the nocebo effect did not go away may be explained by the fact that in the natural world, any stimulus that cues us for pain (and cues our survival instincts) means we should avoid those stimuli. This mechanism of self-protection makes us more susceptible to suggestion when informed by our healthcare providers that they do not have confidence in our ability to give birth vaginally.

When doubt in ourselves takes over, then suddenly the contractions feel more painful, and laboring women start finding reasons to want to escape the birth process. This was very evident in the documentary film *Trial of Labor*. The story followed four women who were seeking a VBAC. Two of the four women who failed to have a VBAC carried the most fear and doubt into their labor. The same two women also had the least amount of emotional support, as depicted by their struggles documented in the film.

Finding Trust in Birth

What are your options when the healthcare provider you decided to trust now suddenly doesn't trust you or your body? First, you have to do your homework and look for providers that have a low C-section rate – less than 15% would be fantastic – and, of course, that are supportive of VBAC's.

Then the next thing you should do is to dig deep inside yourself and find out why it is important for you to have a VBAC. For me, it was all about wanting the most freedom possible in my birth journey. I really wanted to know who I was as a woman. I wanted to have an empowered birth experience. I also wanted my babies to be born in a natural environment.

The birth process brings out your true essence. I knew I had a warrior's heart and needed to prove to myself that I could give birth on my own terms. I didn't want anyone telling me what to do. From the start of all my pregnancies, my goal was to have an out-of-hospital birth, but something always happened that would lead to a transfer to the hospital.

Then my third baby was planned at a hospital with my dear friend and colleague as my midwife and the baby ends up being a surprise breech despite being head down the day before! I still remember the doctor coming into the labor room and saying, "I'm sorry, we'll have to do a C-section, because honestly, I can count on one hand how many breech deliveries I have ever done." What do you say to that? It's a rock and a hard place for sure.

I was 8 to 9 centimeters and really needed to push. I had just gotten an epidural. If I hadn't, I think I would have just pushed the baby out, because I was progressing quickly. Instead, they wheeled me off to the operating room to get a C-section. The entire time, I had a strong urge to push, so much so that I kept telling them to look under the sheets because I really felt like the baby was between my legs.

Despite my pleading, my son was born via C-section, I heard him cry, and the next I knew, I was in recovery. Apparently after the birth they had to heavily sedate me because I was complaining of too much pain while they were closing me up.

I remember having a dream that I was at a campfire with a group of boys roasting marshmallows and telling ghost stories. My family has always been in Boys Scouts, so a dream like that is no surprise. But then

I woke up, and found myself on a stretcher. I reached down to feel for my belly and it was gone.

It was like one of those horror movie moments when the main character realizes her baby is gone. I started crying out for my baby until they finally brought him to me. When I held him, I realized, oh no, I really did have a C-section.

My only consolation was that he was ok, and so was I. But through the years, I had to heal the loss of my natural birth experience. Ironically, if it weren't for that birth journey, I wouldn't be writing this book now. I love my "heads-up" birth journey baby. I learned a lot – specially to make sure you find a provider who is comfortable delivering breech babies!

Partnering to Enhance Relaxation

The next important thing to do is really learn the art of relaxation. When the mind believes that something bad is going to happen in the body, it tends to manifest. The true power of understanding the concepts of the placebo versus the nocebo effects is in knowing that you actually can control your responses during labor and how to receive the information people give you.

Partnering with a positive caregiver is essential, too. A study conducted by Harvard researcher Ted Kaptchuk found that even when subjects were told they'd been given a placebo to treat illness, they still got better as long as they felt nurtured and cared for.

In other words, all you need is the power of your own body and mind and the nurturing care of a healthcare provider knowledgeable about normal birth. Usually, that would be a midwife, because they are trained extensively in the normal birth process and how to respond to emergencies. Using the exercises in this book is also important to help train your mind and body connection to allow the birth to progress easily.

Birth is not an easy process to go through alone, so it makes a big difference if your care provider is also holding the belief that you will be successful at having a vaginal birth too. One of the most important qualities of your birth healthcare provider is that they are forces of healing and not forces of fear or pessimism.

The relationship you have with your birth attendant matters, too, and this is why. Your mind and your perception communicate with your brain. Your brain then communicates with all the cells of the body via hormones and neurotransmitters. So, for example, if you have a negative thought, belief, or feeling coming from your mind, the amygdala part of the brain thinks your survival is being threatened. And it turns on the hypothalamus that talks to the pituitary gland, which then communicates with the adrenal glands and they start spitting out stress hormones like cortisol, norepinephrine, and epinephrine. This cascade of natural biochemicals has now turned on the stress response, coined by Walter Cannon at Harvard in 1915.

Your stress response triggers the **sympathetic nervous system** and puts you into a fight, flight, or freeze mode. This is very adaptive and protective if you are running from a wild animal, but not very effective in labor. The same chemicals activated by the stress response also **stop your uterus from contracting**. Without contractions, labor slows down and may even stop or not even start at all.

In everyday life, you are supposed to have a quick stress response if there is a threat and then it's supposed to switch off. Unfortunately, it does not happen this way. One study showed that, on average, we have more than 50 stressors per day. And if you add feelings of isolation, depression, pessimism, or unhappiness, that number may double.

There is an **antidote to all of this**. The counterbalance for the stress response is the relaxation response described by Herbert Benson, also at Harvard, in 1975. The best part is you can practice and turn on the relaxation response way before labor begins. When you are able to effortlessly engage your relaxation response, then you will be able to turn off your stress response. The **parasympathetic system** of the brain will turn on, and the **healing and birth hormones** like oxytocin, dopamine, nitric oxide, and endorphins fill the body and bathe every cell.

Important: these natural self-care and repair mechanisms can only flip on when the nervous system is relaxed. Getting to the point where you can control the on and off switch takes practice so that you can use this skill from the very start of labor.

This relaxation response is what researchers think explains the placebo effect. The combination of the mind's positive belief and the presence of a nurturing birth healthcare provider help the nervous system relax. In turn, the natural hormones that help start labor and help labor to progress are then released into your body. You will learn how to practice the relaxation techniques that I teach my clients later in the book.

*****

Matrix Reimprinting Your Future Birth Exercise

A good exercise to do now would be to sit back in a comfortable chair, listen to an instrumental piece of music, close your eyes, and use the thumb and index fingers of one hand to gently squeeze the fingertips of your other hand. For best results, have your partner read this to you so that you can fully engage in this process.

While you are doing this, take three slow deep breaths and imagine what the day of your labor will be like. Just make up a story about where you want to be and what you want to be doing when your labor starts.

Now imagine you are going to call your partner to let them know that you think you are in labor. Now you will just patiently wait for your partner to come home from work and, while you are waiting, you decide you will catch up on the laundry and watch comedy movies on TV.

When your partner comes home, you let them know that you think your labor started. Imagine having dinner together. Maybe you decide to go out to eat, or maybe you call for food to be delivered to you.

Now imagine the next part of your labor. The surges and rushes of your contractions are getting much stronger now. If you are having a home birth, you call your midwife and let her know what is happening.

While you wait for her, you decide to get into a warm bath. You have all that you need to help you in labor, including aromatherapy bath salts to help with the contractions. Your partner is at your side, the lights are low, and you have your favorite labor music playlist on.

While you are in the bathtub, your midwife and her assistant arrive. She checks on your baby's heartbeat, and all is well. Time passes, and you are using all the techniques that you have learned from this book to get you through all the contractions. Suddenly, your water breaks and you start to have a strong urge to push.

Now imagine having pushed your baby out. Everything went smoothly. You can see your future self very clearly sitting in bed and nursing your baby. Now I want you to freeze everyone in that picture and say hello to your future self who just had a vaginal delivery at home.

Let her know you are the part of her in the past that is still pregnant. Ask her to tell you the most important thing that you in the present moment can do to ensure that your present self has this wonderful, natural, vaginal birth outcome. Also ask her how she is feeling having had the baby at home.

Listen to what she says and thank her for the advice. If what she said was positive and her feeling is positive, place your hands over your heart and imagine those beautiful positive feelings and advice coming into your body through the top of your head.

Let those beautiful feelings run through all the neuro pathways of your body, into every cell of your body and all the way down to your DNA. Let those positive feelings reach all the way down to your toes and bring them back up through the muscle fibers of your uterus, all the way into your heart.

Let your heart be filled with the positive advice, feelings, and vision of your future self having given a natural vaginal birth. When your heart is full of this beautiful imagery and the uplifting emotions of having given birth vaginally, breathe it all out into the universe, putting into place all the synergy you will need to achieve this goal through all of time, space, and place. You can now gently open your eyes and bring your attention back into the room.

If at any point during this exercise you were not able to reach a positive outcome – in other words, you were not able to see the birth of your dreams – then stop the matrix visualization process and write down what came up. You do not want to imprint negative thoughts or images. Instead, acknowledge them by taking notes. Later in the book, I will be teaching you how to resolve negative emotions and imagery regarding your birth experiences.

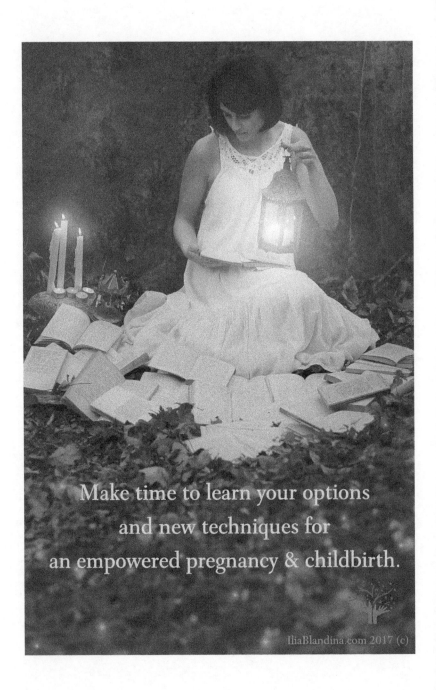

Make time to learn your options
and new techniques for
an empowered pregnancy & childbirth.

IliaBlandina.com 2017 (c)

CHAPTER 5

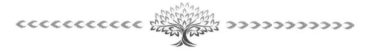

Things They
Don't Teach You

"The truth will set you free. But first, it will piss you off."
~ GLORIA STEINEM

Good News Bad News

Okay, this chapter is about the good news and the bad news of childbirth in the U.S. First I will cover the "bad news" – the kind of stuff that does not get discussed in mainstream childbirth education classes – and then I will end on the "good news" ... that is also not discussed in mainstream childbirth education classes!

The number of American women giving birth by cesarean section is at an all-time high. So, high cesarean sections have now become the most common major surgical procedure performed on women.

49

Unfortunately, maternity care in the United States is in a crisis. Since 1996, the cesarean rate in the U.S. has risen upwards of 46%. Currently, one out of three babies are delivered by a C-section. According to *Consumer Reports,* that is an increase of 500% since 1970!

We will review the history of obstetrics over the past couple of centuries in order to give you an overview of how we got into the problem of over using cesarean sections for birth. Beforehand, let me start by explaining the modern roles of obstetricians, midwives, and doulas.

The Differences Between OB, Midwife, and Doula

An obstetrician (from the Latin "stand before") is frequently a gynecologist as well. They are medical doctors and surgeons who specialize in caring for women, especially those with complicated pregnancies and gynecological problems requiring surgery.

During labor, they specifically monitor for signs of abnormalities and take action via interventions that may include induction of labor, surgical vaginal deliveries with episiotomies, vacuum-assisted deliveries, forceps-assisted deliveries, or major abdominal surgery via a cesarean section.

There are many reasons why all of these interventions may be appropriate, but this book is not designed to discuss that. These discussions are best done face to face with your personal healthcare provider.

Midwives (the word's original meaning was "with woman") have successfully completed a nationally accredited midwifery education program. They are recognized through certification programs as responsible and accountable professionals who work in partnership with women to give necessary care and advice during pregnancy, labor, childbirth, and afterwards during the postpartum period, including general gynecological care and contraceptive management. Midwives work in a variety of settings that may include the home, a birth center, or a hospital.

There are various types of professional midwives, depending on the program they have studied and whether they had been a Registered Nurse before studying and certifying for the title of Midwife. All work independently from a physician when caring for women who are low- to moderate-risk.

A doula is a trained and experienced professional who provides continuous physical, emotional, informational, and practical support to the mother before, during, and just after birth. Doulas do not medically manage your pregnancy or birth, whereas midwives do independently medically manage your pregnancy and deliver your baby.

Obstetrical History in America

In 1715, New York City became the first place to license midwives, who were viewed as servants of the state. They were good at what they did. Death during childbirth was not well-recorded, but at least one historian estimated that the live birth rate at that time was at a healthy 95 percent.

Midwives were crucial because men didn't attend childbirth – it was considered "indecent." Also, there were very few doctors around, and those who weren't well-educated. Surprisingly, doctors weren't required to pass an examination until 1760 – 45 years after midwives were required to be licensed!

In 1765, in Philadelphia, Dr. William Shippen opened the first formal training for midwives. Few attended, because midwives believed that childbirth is a normal process and inherently within the domain of female competence, and questioned the logic of learning from men. Men, however, thought women to be intellectually incapable of learning because they were too emotional. The gender wars evolved into a belief among well-to-do families that a physician could provide better care than female midwives. This gave rise to America becoming the only developed industrialized country to *not* bring midwives into the hospitals.

Interestingly obstetricians and midwives lived up to their named professions. Obstetricians tended "to stand before" women as an authority not to be questioned, while midwives continued the art of being "with woman" by approaching birth as a normal life event and trusting the woman's body to know what to do.

As time went on with the advance of technology, obstetricians got in the habit of mechanizing birth and introducing interventions to make all women fit the same mold. Midwives continued to hold space for women to trust themselves in the birth process, knowing that every birth is different even for the same woman. They also continued to be experts in what is normal in the birth process and therefore able to differentiate if something is going wrong and then provide intervention.

Culture around birth started to change drastically when ether was first used for pain relief in 1848 for humanitarian reasons in Boston by Dr. Walter Channing. Meanwhile, in the early 1900s, physicians started a smear campaign against midwives. They made posters showing a black granny midwife delivering a baby in a very poor home with the racist, misogynistic caption, "Would you want this kind of person to deliver your baby?"

This cultural shift in which midwives were portrayed as a vestige of the old country – dirty, ignorant, illiterate – made it possible for hospitals to stand in contrast as this gleaming, wonderful place where birth would be cleaner and safer. The reality was that giving birth with an obstetrician at that time was much more dangerous than giving birth with a midwife, because many doctors graduating from medical school had not witnessed a live birth before setting out to practice medicine.

OB/GYN specialty hospitals started to sprout up and the business and economics of birth took over. All of a sudden, the concept of "normal" was warped to benefit those in power.

The drug scopolamine (also known as twilight sleep) was invented in Germany in the early 1900s. When American women found out about it, they started demanding for the drug to be used because, after all, "I am a modern woman."

At that time, women were still being told the pain of childbirth was the curse of Eve and unavoidable. But the liberated feminist attitude of the time was that suffering should have nothing to do with childbirth. Women thought the drug took away pain during childbirth, but it didn't and doesn't. It actually just wipes out any memory of the experience. But that did not stop scopolamine's widespread use across the United States. By the 1960's, almost everyone was having twilight sleep.

While this drug took away memory and not the pain, it also took away self-control and self-awareness. Women would scream and try to climb the walls, spit in people's faces, and claw the faces of the doctors and the nurses.

The hospitals ended up strapping women to the hospital beds, using lamb's wool in order to not leave marks on their wrists that would lead their husbands to question what was going on. So essentially, women were strapped to beds and left there for days, sometimes in their own poop and pee. It was a horrible period in American birthing history.

Because of twilight sleep and woman having to be strapped down, the lithotomy position (lying on your back with your legs in stirrups) and birth via forceps became the standard birthing procedure. Even as twilight sleep went out of fashion, the lithotomy position has prevailed and is the most physiologically dysfunctional position ever invented for birth.

Putting the mother flat on her back literally makes the pelvis smaller; makes it much more difficult for the woman to use her stomach muscles to push. Therefore, it makes it much more likely that an episiotomy will be cut and forceps or a vacuum extractor used.

The use of twilight sleep meant mothers were still asleep after giving birth since they were exhausted from the labor and were still under the effects of the medication. Worse, the babies were also under the effect of the medication, because it had crossed the placenta. Babies' ability to breathe was affected, and they needed close monitoring for hours after birth. Thus, the newborn nursery came about, as well as the development of formula and bottle feeding. The medication also showed up in breast milk, so breastfeeding was discouraged under the guise that formula feeding was better for the baby. (Shh, don't tell them it was the drugs given during labor; they don't need to know that.) Remember, what you don't know might still hurt you or your baby.

Trial and Error Obstetrics

In the past century, obstetrics basically has been used as a live trial to practice whatever new methods were invented at the time without considering potential bad outcomes. In the 1930s, they were performing x-rays on every pregnant woman to measure her pelvis. And then in the 1940s, they discovered x-rays caused the babies to have cancer. So, they had to stop.

In the 1950s and 60s, they used a drug called thalidomide. It was marketed to a world hooked on tranquilizers and sleeping pills post-WWII as an over-the-counter sleep aid and motion sickness remedy, but was found to cause babies to be born without arms and legs, so they had to stop that, too.

In every case, harmful practices were halted only after the damage was done.

In the 1990s, they were giving Cytotec to induce labor in women who had a previous cesarean. At the time, medical schools were trying to develop a low-cost form of labor induction they could introduce to underdeveloped countries that could not afford Pitocin and the IV pumps needed for its administration.

An interesting fact is Cytotec (misoprostal) is a medication used for ulcers in the intestines, and the FDA classifies it as a category X drug in the Physicians' Desk Reference (PDR) because it causes the abortion of your pregnancy. Yes, they were using it for its off-label effects – in other words, not as it was intended. What they ended up with were hundreds and hundreds of ruptured uteruses and many dead babies before they found out finally, in 1999, that they shouldn't use that medication for women with a previous cesarean. This is what started the pendulum to swing towards having no VBACs at all.

The doctors did not want to admit it was the medication. Blaming it on the client's history of a cesarean was more convenient and protective for them. A repeat C-section was easier to schedule than waiting for natural labor to start. It created a more convincing argument to not have a trial of labor.

Essentially, history shows a complete lack of careful study of the long-term effects of medications and other obstetric interventions before introduction to the public. Therefore, if you really want a humanized birth, the best thing to do is to get the hell out of the hospital or at least be very selective about the hospital you choose to give birth in. Find out their cesarean section rate in advance.

The Emergence of Natural Childbirth

The natural childbirth movement was sparked by and was a reaction against the abuses of the scopolamine era, because some people realized that the only way to get away from that was to get out of the hospital altogether. The home birth movement grew at a good pace again after being basically eliminated at the turn of the 20th century.

It became very popular during the hippie era, when there were communes. These intentional communities mimicked in many ways the kind of immigrant communities, with their extended families, that had existed in the past. Women wanted choices. They didn't want someone else making the rules; especially people who did not understand them. Hospitals were treating women like machines instead of people with feelings. The proponents of home birth knew that this affected birth. They wanted freedom to give birth in whatever position or environment they felt most comfortable in. Midwives were popular again.

But while the home birth scene was burgeoning, so was technology. In 1970, the electronic fetal monitor was introduced into hospitals, and by the end of the decade it was pervasive in hospital births. Interestingly, the cesarean rate in that decade went from 4% to 23%. Much of this was due to false interpretation of fetal heart rate distress patterns, which were actually caused by interventions during labor.

Immediately after an epidural, maternal blood pressure can drop. That, combined with the effects of the medication, causes changes in the fetal heart rate that mimic distress. An epidural may also cause labor to slow down, because you are given large amounts of intravenous hydration to help prevent the low blood pressure in the first place. Also remember if a woman is low-risk, her blood pressure may be naturally low to begin with. It all becomes a vicious cycle of chasing the side effects of interventions.

The modern medical profession has convinced the vast majority of women that they don't know how to give birth. It has also encouraged women to believe that not only are they "too posh to push," but that they are safer with a "designer birth" experience: picking the date and having an elective C-section for no medical or obstetrical reason whatsoever.

Much of this came about for monetary and legal reasons, not because it is the best choice for the mother and the baby. In fact, as soon as a midwife's practice reached more than 30% of the women in a certain hospital, the doctors would fire her or rescind any agreement to back her up for emergencies. In this way, the perceived competition could be illuminated. Or insurance companies would not reimburse her with the claim that there were enough providers in the county giving OB care.

Interesting facts:

- In 1900, 95% of births in the United States took place at home
- In 1938, half of all births took place at home
- By 1955, less than 1% of births took place at home
- It remains that number today

The majority of the time, women have uneventful, normal labor and births. But current hospital protocols and systems that demand you stay in bed, hooked up to monitors and unable to eat, walk around, or do whatever you want can prevent normal, uneventful births from occurring. If you really have a goal of a natural birth, keep in mind that the odds are greater for having unnecessary interventions and a higher chance of a C-section at the hospital.

Natural Birth Bait and Switch

Most women are told through advertising or prenatal classes that are given at the hospitals to "come to us, we'll take care of everybody's birth, doesn't matter what kind of birth you want, we are open to anything." And then you get there, and you realize, no, the hospital system is really set up one way: to handle one kind of birth, and you just get put through their system and bound by their rules. It becomes a fight to try to *not* get put through that system.

Another standard is that in hospitals, you are not allowed to have very long labors. So, if you are not dilating rapidly, which you are likely not to do if you get an epidural early in labor, you will be given Pitocin by IV.

Pitocin makes contractions longer, stronger, and closer together. And that makes the pain of labor much worse. After a while, the epidural may start to lose its effectiveness. Eventually the pain of the contractions overwhelms the epidural, and you need to increase the epidural. This may cause labor to slow down again, so you need more Pitocin. It becomes a vicious cycle of using each drug to counterbalance the effect of the other one.

You're not feeling the pain of the heavy contractions, because your epidural is higher. The extra Pitocin is causing your baby to get more compressed. The Pitocin contractions are so long and strong that the blood and oxygen flow to the baby may be compromised. So then, the baby is likely to go into distress, which means you'll be sent off for an emergency cesarean for a baby in distress, which is caused by the contractions induced by the Pitocin, which was necessitated by the epidural. Remember, what you don't know might still hurt you or your baby.

In the hospital, about 90% of patients are on some type of labor augmentation at some point. If you are not making progress in a certain period of time, then the protocol says it's time to facilitate things. Ah! Give me natural labor any day.

Also, what everyone forgets to take into account is the innate stress response that kicks in when a woman changes her environment while in labor. This is bound to happen when a woman and her partner think they are in labor and decide it's time to go either to the birth center or the hospital.

If you are in early, instead of true active labor (defined as being 6 centimeters dilated), then chances are that a change in your physical surroundings will slow down your labor and may even stop it all together. You can prevent this from happening simply by having your baby at home with a midwife specializing in home birth. Your next best option is a birth center, but depending on your state of residence, they may not be allowed to do a VBAC there, so you will have to research that.

Birth centers are more forgiving if you have a false alarm and your labor stops after you arrive. When you arrive at a hospital, however, it will all depend on who is on call and their philosophy. Some practitioners will not let you leave, and you may not warm up to the idea of having to stay in bed and be monitored the whole time. These are all things to research and discuss with your healthcare provider.

The best thing you can do if you are low-risk is to learn how to manage your response to the early labor contractions at home so that you can stay home as long as possible. Low-risk essentially means you don't have any risk factors that require monitoring during labor in addition to the history of having a cesarean. In other words, if you only have a history of having a previous C-section, then you are essentially low-risk.

The bottom line is that hospitals are businesses. They want those beds filled and emptied. They don't want women hanging around in the labor room. That's why one intervention leads to a series of interventions, and the result is that the mother finally ends up with cesarean and everyone says, "Thank God, we were able to do all those interventions to save your baby."

The reality is that if they didn't start the cascade of interventions, none of that would have been necessary. Induction of labor has been clearly associated with an increased risk of needing a cesarean delivery.

What You Don't Know Might Still Hurt You or Your Baby

When you look at obstetrics in general, there's been a series of very intense interventions that physicians have been doing day in and day out to millions of women, and there is not a medically justified reason for doing so. The general public doesn't have this information. One of the big problems in this country is the information that is given to women – or the lack thereof.

Common sense tells me that positioning a woman in labor on her back with her legs up forces her into a position that is neither the most comfortable nor the most logical to give birth. This position is better for the doctor, but it makes it nearly impossible for the baby to come out naturally.

There really is not an informed consent obtained from women. No one talks about all of the downsides, all of the things that can go wrong in a C-section, or that the risks of a vaginal delivery are fewer than with a C-section. And what a lot of people don't know is that a C-section is major surgery. The literature is very clear that having a vaginal birth is statistically the best way to go, even after having a cesarean with a previous birth. But women are not being guided towards that.

For almost everyone, the first C-section is fairly simple. It's the second, the third, the fourth, and the fifth C-section that pose a huge risk to the mom in terms of injury to her bladder, injury to the intestines and long-term gynecologic issues in the future such as chronic pelvic pain due to excessive internal scar tissue.

In my role as a midwife, I have performed first assist on many C-section deliveries. I've had patients where there are massive amounts of scar tissue that have formed on the bladder and loops of bowel wrapped around the uterus (due to previous deliveries), and the surgeon has to cut through all that before we can even get to the baby. There may be blood loss that can't necessarily be controlled. It's major surgery, and yet nowadays C-sections are presented like it's a spa day – and bonus, you have a baby!

Another thing not being discussed is that there are many women with C-sections that end up with really bad infections, and those infections are becoming harder to treat with antibiotics. This is one area where I feel like we are regressing in our medical advances, because having an infection that you cannot treat is awful – and the risk of that happening is getting higher.

"Most of the deaths that do take place in the United States
happen for women who went to the hospital, how do I know
that? Because half a percentage of women give birth at home,
and yet our death rate is higher than some third world countries.
We have areas in the United States where it's sky high."

~ INA MAY GASKIN CPM

EXECUTIVE DIRECTOR OF THE FARM BIRTH CENTER

It's sad to say, but people in our culture spend more time and effort researching options for buying a computer, a surround sound system, a car, a camera, or a cell phone than they do checking out what their choices are for birth. We talk about giving mothers options, but what isn't talked about is the degree to which options are being closed off.

One example is birth centers. Since their inception in New York 1975, they have been hard to find and have been in an economic battle with hospitals ever since they began. Of course, hospitals do not say it is based on economics; instead the hospitals make it a challenge for birth centers by blocking hospital privileges to Nurse Midwives who run the birth centers and by politically challenging the birth centers licensure, or even withholding advanced agreement for medical back-up for a transfer. This means that many birth centers or home birth specialist have to rely on whoever is on call at the hospital for obstetrics without knowing in advance the quality of their back-up.

Hospital staff culture also look down at clients that need a transfer into the hospital, feeling like they are about to inherit a "train wreck" of medical mismanagement. The good news is there have been two studies now showing the benefits of delivering at birth centers. Both were done by The American Association of Birth Centers and are called The National Birth Center Study I & II. The first study looked at birth outcomes from 1985 – 1987 and the second from 2007 -2010. The study found that 9 out of 10 women who entered labor *planning* a birth center birth achieved a vaginal delivery. In other words, the C-section rate for these low-risk women was 6 % compared to the U.S. C-section rate of 32%.

Maybe you were told the C-section you had was done because your baby was too big to deliver vaginally. This is one of the most common reasons why elective first C-sections are performed. It's like a pre-emptive strike to try to avoid shoulder dystocia (the baby's shoulders getting stuck under the pubic bone).

What they don't tell you is that there can be a shoulder dystocia during a C-section that may even require a vacuum-assisted delivery, and that a shoulder dystocia can happen even with small babies. Also, an ultrasound can only predict the weight of your baby at + or – 500 grams. That's a one-pound margin of error!

The largest baby I personally attended as a midwife in delivery weighed 11 lbs. It was the mom's first baby, and while it took a while for her to push him out – about three hours – she did it without an episiotomy or a tear. We had to be creative in her pushing positions, but she was able to do it naturally.

In my experience, if the baby is moving down with each push, it will fit through the pelvis. And if the shoulders have been tight, there are gentle maneuvers that midwives know will help guide the baby out safely.

J.W. Williams, the author of *Williams Obstetrics*, the top-selling textbook on obstetrics in history, wrote about vaginal births back when C-section was an emergency operation, done only under the direst circumstances. When writing specifically about C-sections, he put it this way:

> *"Cesarean section requires only a few minutes of time and a modicum of operative experience: while vaginal birth often implies active mental exertion, many hours of patient observation, and frequently very considerable technical dexterity."*
>
> ~ JOHN WHITRIDGE WILLIAMS
> PIONEER OF ACADEMIC OBSTETRICS

As you can see, even the father of academic obstetrics felt that knowing how to attend a woman during a vaginal birth was a highly-acquired skill, one that midwives are the most skilled at performing. Cesarean sections were never meant to replace vaginal birth. The problem now is, if we don't prepare our minds as well as our bodies for birth, this, combined with the general inattention to the cesarean trend, runs a greater risk that C-sections will replace normal vaginal birth.

Is Birth About Control?

Is the nature of birth really something that needs to be controlled or is it something that we need to let go of and just let happen? I think both are important. *The way you can "control birth" is by getting all the information you need* in order to choose the best options for you and your family. *In the end, it's all about the letting go*, so part of the preparation is doing exercises that help you *relax into the labor process and let go of all concerns*. Therefore, it's essential to do your homework and practice these techniques far in advance of the first contraction.

The option of a home birth is very reasonable if you are low risk, even if you have had a C-section before. Your healthcare provider can help you determine your personal risk factors.

I believe that women who choose homebirth have something in common. It might just be a feeling that they know how they want to do things. I think when they are in labor, they are able to interact with their birth journey in different ways. One of which is being surrounded by the people who will support their decisions instead of making decisions for them. In this choice, they also have the added benefit of being able to stay in the same location and not be affected by the stress of traveling to a different location while in active labor.

As humans, we have the gift of free will and choice. Don't let anyone take that from you. The choice of how you want to give birth after C-section is your true power and basic human right. Making up stories and allowing fear to take over undermines your purpose of experiencing life as it should be experienced.

Body-Mind Quantum Connection in Birth

The body-mind is interactive, and we must look at consciousness as it relates to the function of our physical body through birth. Quantum mechanics came into play during the 20th century. One of the concepts is that consciousness itself is a non-local phenomenon. What that means is that in consciousness, we are unified everywhere and every when. It is our focus of attention or our alignment, as well as what we pay attention to at any single moment, that create our reality.

Right now, I am paying attention to being in the body. But that does not mean I don't exist everywhere and every when. Matter comes out of mind instead of mind coming out of matter. All particles and all things have these dual components of local manifestation and non-local existence. So perhaps by observing our physical bodies, we can identify the non-localness of who we are. What we end up learning is that existence and information is not only the basis of our being but also our knowing. Stay with me; it will make sense by the end.

Spirit is the fundamental vibration of nothing. But by "nothing," I mean the absolute void from which everything comes. Similar to what happens at conception, spirit is the unseen world of life itself. Mind, consciousness and this mysterious spiritual essence of who we are does not have space-time coordination. This is why the exercise of visualizing the birth you want in advance is a very effective way of birth planning.

We can't scientifically prove any of this stuff of course, and that's where anyone who is scientifically or rationally minded will dismiss this – because if it is not scientifically proven, then it doesn't exist. What you need to take into consideration is that there are many things we do in life that have not been scientifically proven.

For example, there is a lot of anecdotal evidence right now about near-death experiences and out-of-body experiences. It's so prevalent that there is a department in the military that studies remote viewing (seeing things that are happening from far away) as part of our national defense system. There are children being born with detailed memories of relatives who have died years before the child was born. There are many cases of reincarnation memories.

These cases have allowed scientists to take quantum physics and explore it in new ways in the last several years. This opens brand new doors that have never been open before in understanding ourselves, understanding the deepest part of our nature, and understanding consciousness itself.

There is a coming together of science and spirituality, and this is important to the birth process. In order to "give birth a chance," you must find your birth journey compass and follow it, instead of letting someone else lead you. This is why the exercise of a future birth reimprinting works. Consciously accessing the "you" that is one of your potential futures is, to some degree, like astral projection or remote viewing your own future.

The ability to tune into your future consciousness and become aware of your innate ability to obtain guidance from the part of you that has a VBAC brings that reality into the present moment. That exercise helps you to connect to the future outcome you desire through the energetic matrix we are in. What we experience in the past or the future is what is being accessed during Matrix Reimprinting.

When trying to understand all of this, the only thing I am asking you to consider is that you are more than your physical body. Tapping on your finger points and visualizing yourself in the future helps to put you into a relaxed state. Once you are there, you begin to open up and expand into the energy that you are. This expansion of your consciousness is more than your physical body.

We've known for years that when we are in that deeply relaxed state, we let go of our defenses. We let go of blocks and obstacles, or bring them to light so we can obtain clarity and resolution. These blocks and obstacles may get in the way of exploring our deepest fears or desires. So from that place of deep relaxation, we can then open up to all kinds of possibilities. Ancient cultures have been doing this through drumming, dance, chanting, and rituals for many thousands of years.

I have also included a link to guided meditations in my VBAC Tool Kit. The meditations use music to guide you into a theta brainwave state, and will allow you to develop an awareness of information and concepts that are not ordinarily available to our waking state. This is a bridge for opening a gateway for the out-of-body experience that is reaching your future self, the one who has experienced the goal of a VBAC.

This is just one piece of a full range of possible experiences that would be useful in helping you to become better able to know your total self before and during your birth journey. My work with clients one on one has helped them gain their own personalized range of possibilities.

Mind over Matter: Quantum Holograms and the Matrix Birth

As women, we need to look past 3D reality. Whether we know it or not, the female mind has the ability to connect to the 4D reality, and that needs to be taught and understood during pregnancy and childbirth. Rest assured "the female mind" is also in men as well.

We are living in a physical body that is alive because of us. We give life to this physical life. Mind exists because we give life to that mind. Without us the physical body would disappear, become dust. What we really are is life, and eternal. It never ends, it never begins, and life is shifting, growing, and forming. There is nothing but transformation.

Think of it like you are looking through the lens of a telescope. If you are looking through it and the image is sharp, that is called being in focus. As you turn the dials, the image starts to get blurry. That is called un-focusing. Now an unfocused image means that the light from the object is going through many different pathways to reach your eyes. So that light is getting to your eyes from different directions all at the same time, and it makes the image appear blurry.

You can apply this analogy to the concept of parallel realities in that they are all happening and you are seeing all the realities at once, instead of focusing on one reality. This process is what we are doing when we learn to focus on a potential future for ourselves. We start by learning new things and as we do, we begin to let go of old ways of thinking that no longer serve us. We then are able to learn new things that better serve us and our goals. This is the process of life.

Life is still the great mystery. What is really going on? What is it that survives? The work of the Institute of Noetic Science has shown that information survives. The information survives in holographic form. Nature preserves information in a quantum hologram that becomes a record of our life.

Ancient lore acknowledges this as well and they call it the Akashic Record, as mentioned in Chapter 1. The Akashic Record is the record of life, and was recognized by ancient cultures. The Institute of Noetic Sciences is now starting to see that. They call it the Zero Point Energy

Field, also known as the quantum hologram, and is the equivalent of the Akashic Record.

The quantum hologram is based on the fact that matter emits and reabsorbs a quantum of energy and photons at the most basic level of nature. These photons have a non-local interconnection regardless of where they go, therefore, they are always interconnected. Information is stored as energy at the smallest level of existence, and can be retrieved if you learn how to focus your mind on it. This fundamental discovery essentially explains how information at the quantum level of nature is as important as energy itself.

What the physicists tell us is that when particles are entangled, they maintain a correlation and a coherence. If something happens to one particle, it is instantaneously known or recognized by the other particle – regardless of where they are in the universe. That is instantaneous communication, and it is called non-locality. How would one experience that personally? By using matrix reimprinting to communicate with the future reality you want.

This instant communication that you had with your future self and the imprinting of what it feels like to have a successful VBAC into your present body is how you were able to use the concept of non-locality. By communicating with the future self that has a VBAC, you are creating entangled particles that maintain a correlation with your present reality and your life.

You are in the habit of feeling yourself in this body. But when you become non-locally aware by communicating with the future self that experiences a successful VBAC, you learn that perhaps you are more than your body. This allows you to become aware of information that you are not aware of through your physical senses. Instead, the information and guidance is available only if you are non-locally communicating with your successful future self. By the same token, you can communicate with your past self and heal the negative emotional impact of specific events.

The exercise of using the quantum holograms of the matrix energy field that surrounds us helps us to connect with feelings that we couldn't know with our senses. When that information comes to us, we are able to transform it into positive feelings that change our present lives. This ability of being able to access information that is non-local is considered to be a way to understand the nature of the real reality that we are in. And it can be used every day.

In the exercise, you read at the end of Chapter 4, you saw one of the ways I help my clients access their potential for having a successful VBAC. My clients learn how to access an alternate reality of themselves that before was made invisible by their fears of failing and the events of their past. This is done by first healing the basis of their fears, and then going into the future and imprinting into their present reality the feeling of being successful and safe in their birth journey.

*****

Stress Release Exercise Using "Right Brain Start-Up"

That was a lot of information! So let me teach you a self-regulating exercise that you can do any time you feel overwhelmed. Before you begin, have a glass of water nearby. Now follow these steps:

- First, relax back into your chair.
- Make three simple physical movements to get yourself comfortable.
- Now take three sips of water.
- Relax back into your chair and take three gentle breaths.

Inhale through your nose and exhale through your mouth. You can even sigh while you are exhaling. Try to exhale longer than your inhale, and with each breath, fill your lungs a little more each time. Remember to breathe from your diaphragm by letting your lower abdomen expand as opposed to only expanding your upper chest. You can place your hands on your lower belly so that you become aware of it expanding with each inhale and contracting with each exhale.

From this place of quiet contemplation and relaxation do the following:

- Notice three things – one in your immediate external environment, one in your physical body, and one in your emotional state. Just be a sacred witness to these three states of being, and then let them float away.
- Now I want you to think of three things you are grateful for in your outside world that happened in the last week. Let the gratitude float around you like thank you bubbles.
- Now think of three things you are grateful for about yourself. They may be things that you accomplished in the last week, or any self-care that you made time for.
- Finish by spending the next three minutes in silence, sending love to your baby, visualizing what it is like to be your baby inside of you, and holding your baby in a state of love and gratitude for joining you in your life journey.

Adapted from *Right Brain Start Up,* © Sandra H. Rodman, www.RightBrainAerobics.com, used with permission.

When you are ready, open your eyes, start moving your body, stretch, drink some water, have a snack, and I will meet you in the next chapter!

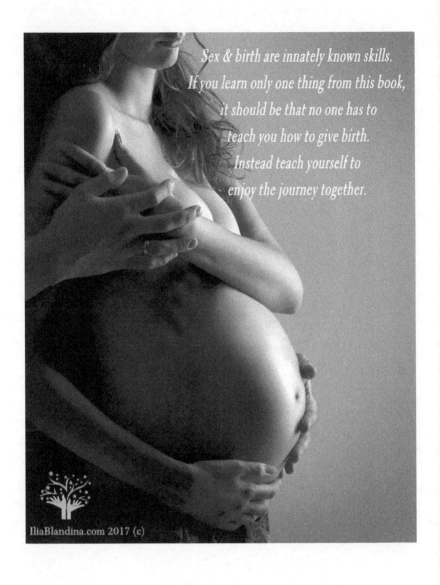

Sex & birth are innately known skills.
If you learn only one thing from this book,
it should be that no one has to
teach you how to give birth.
Instead teach yourself to
enjoy the journey together.

CHAPTER 6

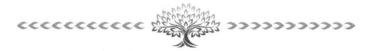

A Passionate Birth

"A woman is the full circle.
Within her is the power to create, nurture and transform."
~ DIANE MARIECHILD

Sex and Birth

When we cultivate a rapport with our sexual partner that is based on the desire to share pleasure and exploration, we can carry this dynamic of sharing into our birth journey. This experience of mutual pleasure during labor awakens the bliss centers in the brain, and opens us up to joy, love, and mystical experiences during birth.

The brain regions activated during orgasm are the amygdala and the hypothalamus, which produces oxytocin, the hormone needed to start and maintain uterine contraction during labor and birth. This is also the love and bonding hormone. Oxytocin levels jump fourfold during an orgasm.

One of the best things to do if you think you are near labor is to make love with your partner. Not only will you have oxytocin levels working for you, but the prostaglandins in semen also help promote uterine contractions and soften your cervix. There's an old saying: *"It took love to put the baby in your belly, it will take love to get the baby out."*

The birth journey is an incredibly important experience for women, and yet they have been told for years that they are not responsible for their own birth process. **If you learn only one thing from this book, it should be that no one has to teach you how to give birth.** It is an innate knowing. The most important thing you can do is clear out the clutter of fearful thoughts that have been implanted by the media and modern western medicine. Your passionate birth journey and the key to unlocking it are already in your body.

They Have No Idea What Birth Is

Today most obstetricians have no idea what a birth can really be like. How do I know this? Because the C-section rate is steadily climbing. Very few doctors have ever observed a normal birth while in medical school or in the hospital.

All they usually see are vaginal births shrouded by epidurals, Pitocin inductions, and sections. If you were to ask any medical student if they have seen a fully natural birth, most would answer "rarely" or "almost never." The best chance for them to see natural birth would be if midwives were a part of their education, and the chance of that happening is decreasing.

Some attending physicians don't even see the point of trying to have a natural birth. Dr. Michael Brodman, Chairman of the OB/GYN department at Mount Sinai Hospital in New York said in the documentary, *The Business of Being Born*, *"I call it 'feminist machismo,' you know when you are pushing your baby in a stroller three months later, to say 'I did it naturally,' personally I don't think it's important."* There is something going on in how we take care of women during birth when doctors have this kind of outlook about natural birth. It made me cringe when I heard him say that. It is very troubling, especially in the United States.

I believe our healthcare system is badly broken around the perception of natural birth, and it is largely because we have lost respect for and belief in a woman's body to be able to give birth naturally. The medical establishment has become arrogant. They have come to think that with all of the modern technology and all they have learned in the past century, they have mastered nature.

Mind you, as it was revealed in the previous chapter, this modern progress was done through trial and error and at the expense of many lives. Many times, modern obstetricians find it repellent to think that maybe nature could be better than they are.

Trust in the Passion of Birth

And yet natural and passionate birth does happen. When women are educated to trust in their body and to know that giving VBAC birth a chance isn't a taboo, beautiful births happen on their own, without any medical interventions. I have met many obstetricians to whom this idea is a narcissistic wound. They don't know what to do with it, and they dismiss the idea as an uneducated notion, a pipe dream. What they are hiding from their patients is that it makes them feel helpless, hopeless, and useless.

Fortunately, there are some obstetricians that believe in birth. They are needed and are very helpful. Obstetricians and all healthcare providers are essential to the process of healing clients and the system. We need to embrace the idea that love and passion should come first.

Women need to change their outlook as well. We all need to emerge from a state of fear and trauma by moving into a full immersion of love and passion. It's not just the doctors; we as women need to stop thinking that our body is not our business. We need to challenge the belief that the safest way to approach birth is to take our power and hand it over to other healthcare providers.

Our body and birth journey is our business. We need to realize that our mind has tremendous power to communicate with our body. Together, they know how best to arrange our birth journey.

A passionate birth journey is best achieved with natural birth. You will get the highest oxytocin rush you will ever have in your life when you give birth naturally. Many times, women go into an altered state of consciousness and are in a state of bliss. Yes, there is pain, but it gets all entangled together. You cannot have bliss without pain.

When a woman feels safe and supported during birth; her brain releases endorphins that are 18 to 33 times more potent than morphine! This is the intangible essence of the phrase "no pain, no gain" when it comes to labor. But at the same time, given the proper instruction before birth, many women can release the concept of pain as related to birth. In other words, they can change their perception and instead of perceiving pain, they embrace the ebb and flow of contractions as surges of energy and rushes of bliss.

Promoting a passionate birth experience means allowing you to move. The more you move through your contractions, the less intense they feel. Many women find moving their hips during labor is very helpful. Most doctors don't tell women this, but if you are experiencing back pain in labor, the best thing you can do is lean over and swing your hips back and forth.

In fact, I recommend that my clients enroll in beginner belly dance classes, because the basic level one movements help to get your baby in the most desirable position for birth.

One of the ways to prevent back labor in the first place is to always start your evening by lying on your right side. This not only will help you avoid acid reflux from your stomach, but will also help your baby settle into position with the back of its head towards your front right hip. This position makes for a faster labor and delivery. When I practiced at birth centers, I would look for that type of presentation. If it was present, I would advise my clients to call if their membranes break before feeling any contractions because more than likely they would be ready to push within six hours.

When having a passionate birth experience some women may even have orgasms. Oxytocin release, combined with endorphins and an environment where women feel they can be themselves, enables women to relax into the complete process – and orgasms are quite possible.

Touch as Communication

Some women want to be held and touched during labor, and others don't. Either way, by practicing these techniques before labor starts, you will learn which one you may be and how your partner can avoid getting smacked!

Note to your birth partner: When a woman in labor suddenly snaps at you and says, "Don't touch me!" what she really means is "Don't touch me (that way)!" Most women in labor prefer a firm, sure touch rather than feather light, rapid, nervous touching, which will more than likely produce the infamous labor smack!

*****

Touch as Positive Communication

Moms:

- Most like to have their lower back, inner thighs, or the palm of one hand massaged during a contraction.
- Practice all three exercises above with ice (reviewed in Chapter 8), and see which one you like best. (Although that might change when you are in actual labor.)
- During practice audibly exhale so your partner will be able to hear the cue of when to touch you. During labor, this will happen naturally.
- Practice being aware of your breath as well as the sensation of touch.
- Give feedback to your partner as to whether the touch was too soft or too deep, or if the timing was off.

Partners:

- Remember to use a 60-second timer when practicing with ice.
- Pay close attention to her breathing pattern.
- When she exhales, use a "downward" (pressing into her body) stroke and match the length of her exhale.
- Lighten your stroke when she inhales, moving your touch back to the starting point.
- Then stroke "downward" again when she exhales.
- Your touch should mirror the intensity of her breath, both in speed and intensity.
- If her breathing remains too fast or erratic after the peak of the contraction, you can help her breathe more slowly and calmly by gradually slowing down your strokes.

Touch as a Cue to Bring Her Back into Her Body

- Place both your hands over her heart and ask her to breath into your hands.
- Then place both your hands over her solar plexus (top of the belly) and ask her to breathe into your hands again.
- Now place both your hands over her lower belly and ask her to breathe into your hands once more.

*****

The Love Hormone of Bonding

The other function that natural oxytocin release facilitates is bonding with and protecting the baby. Of course, first and foremost, oxytocin travels in the blood stream down to the uterus to start triggering and maintaining the contractions of labor, and that's when the switch to the maternal brain circuits gets turned on. This whole brain cocktail of hormones and neuro transmitters has for millions of years been developed to keep the mommy absolutely focused on the protection of the newborn baby.

One of the things to note about Pitocin is that it is a synthetic version of oxytocin that is used intravenously to start labor or to make labor stronger in hospitals, but it doesn't act as natural oxytocin would in the brain. Sometimes modern medical interventions are necessary, but they also inhibit natural maternal bonding to protect the baby and to nourish the baby right after birth.

Until recently, love was a topic for poets, novelists, and philosophers. Today, it is studied from multiple scientific perspectives. For mammals in general, there is a short period of time immediately after birth that will never happen again and is critical in mom's bonding with their baby.

In order to give birth, a woman, like all mammals, is supposed to release this complex cocktail of love hormones. Immediately after birth, mom and baby both are under the effect of this natural cocktail of oxytocin and endorphins that help create a state of dependency between them.

The synthetic form of these natural chemicals actually does not have the same effect; they instead make both the mom and baby sedated and interfere with the bonding process. When birth occurs naturally and the mother and baby are close to each other, it is the beginning of the attachment process needed to survive. But today, most women give birth without releasing this flow of love hormones. Therefore, the attachment process is being interfered with from the very start of life.

If you disturb the hormonal balance of female mammals giving birth in the wild, the result is simple: the mother does not take care of her baby. Studies have shown that when monkeys give birth by C-section, the mother is not interested in her baby.

So, you wonder, but what about us? If the majority of women are forced into repeat C-sections by either biased informed consent or by banning VBACs, what about the future of humanity? This would mean that most women having babies would not have the opportunity to release this cocktail of love hormones the way it is naturally intended by the body. Can we survive without love? We need to create a new awareness of how sacred and passionate birth is designed to be.

Passion during Home Birth

When I was in labor with my fourth baby, a VBAC at home, I remember my midwife and husband reminding me of all the reasons why I was at home and the gift I was giving our baby. And with each contraction I was one step closer. When it was time to push, I didn't feel ready. First I was afraid I might wake up the other kids, then I was afraid I might scare my midwife's child, who she'd brought to the birth (he had witnessed many births).

I then focused on the time. I had started my labor the evening before his due date, and now it was 20 minutes before midnight. I said, "I will start pushing after midnight." My previous babies were anywhere between one to three weeks late, this time I wanted to be on time! My midwife said, "Sure, if that's what you want, but his head is right here." I said, "That's what I want."

I just let the contractions do the pushing for me until I couldn't hold back any longer. I remember losing all sense of time and space. It was like I was floating above the bed. At a certain point, I just gave into the urge to push. I let go and surrendered into my warrior scream. That's when things went really quickly. Before I knew it, Adam was born. It was so empowering. And it was like: finally, this is what I was after. This is what I wanted for my birth journey and my baby.

The research on home birth is pretty consistent in showing that in a supported environment – with people who are trained and have a backup system and can transfer to the hospital quickly if needed – the outcomes of home births are very good. Consistently at least as good as and generally better than they would be in a hospital birth.

The gist of all the studies is that home birth is safer. Midwives have set guidelines by which they determine whether a woman is a good candidate for home birth. Midwives look at women's medical health history and their previous pregnancies, and then prepare themselves for the possibility of a transfer to the hospital. They are experienced at and ready to make that judgment call.

Some people have this image of a home birth midwife walking into somebody's house with a little towel that they roll up and ask the mother to bite on. The fact of the matter is that they bring all the equipment of a portable hospital. This includes Pitocin just in case there is too much bleeding immediately after birth, oxygen, equipment for suturing, and equipment for resuscitating the baby if necessary. Trained home birth midwives are incredibly skilled at what they do, and they are experts in natural, passionate births.

During all of my personal vaginal births, there were times when I was trying to escape labor in my mind. I remember talking to myself at one point when I was in labor with Adam at home. *"I wonder if it's too late to go to the hospital and get that epidural?"* Then I would answer myself, *"Yep, it's too late, remember you wanted this and now you've got it, you are going to have to figure it out. Look around you, you have all the support you need to make this happen, get it together and do it!"*

Then I thought to myself, "I'm not pushing because it hurts too much," followed by the thought, "Ok, if I don't lean into this I will just stay pregnant forever and be in pain forever." One more contraction passed without pushing, and I thought, "No I will not stay like this forever!" What followed were a few loud warrior woman screams. I remembered the scene from *Braveheart*, when William Wallace, face painted half blue, screamed out just before charging into battle. And that was exactly what I did to make it happen.

Every single woman who is having natural childbirth feels like they want to escape at a certain point. And in that feeling of being stuck between a rock and a hard place, they have to surrender to what their body needs to do. Passion needs to fill every cell of the body.

It's incredible when a woman comes to the end of this journey and she says, "You know, I thought I couldn't do it, and then I did it. I hit a wall that was higher than anything I have ever seen in my life, and I conquered it!" It's the most exciting time in a woman's life, an experience like no other, and it can be the most passionate and adventurous day of her life, too.

It's a day where you go through so much pain and so much emotion, and you know you are alive. In the end, you realize you have experienced the most unique event of your life. You have that natural high that people describe. You just feel so accomplished; nothing compares to this. You realize that *"If I could do that, I could do anything,"* and to me, that is the power of birthing; and that is what we are taking away from women.

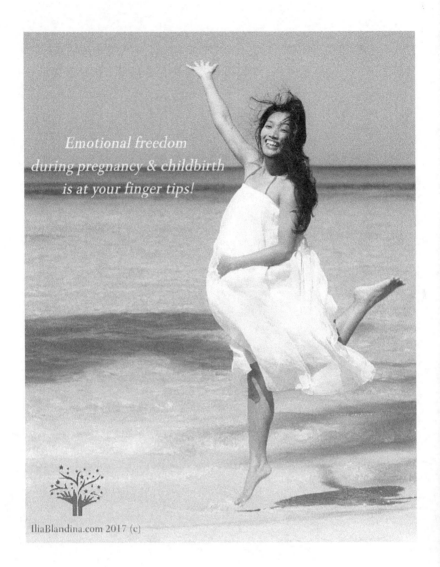

Emotional freedom during pregnancy & childbirth is at your finger tips!

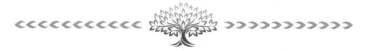

CHAPTER 7

Emotional Freedom

"Instead of resisting any emotion, the best way to dispel it is to enter it fully, embrace it and see through your resistance."
~ DEEPAK CHOPRA

motional freedom: yes, it is possible, doable, and obtainable. Freedom from the crazy rollercoaster of negative emotions about the memory of your previous birth or the anticipatory fear of your next birth – it's all within your reach, quite literally at the tip of your fingers! The secret is, you have to do the work before you go into labor. I hear you: "What, I have to labor before I labor?" Sort of. Let me explain the mechanics of how you can have emotional freedom by using EFT.

What Is EFT?

Emotional Freedom Techniques (EFT), also called tapping, is a stress reduction and relaxation tool that uses the meridian points discovered over 5000 years ago in the healing modality of acupuncture. EFT is part of the field of energy psychology, and was developed by Stanford-trained engineer and performance coach Gary Craig.

Instead of needles, EFT uses tapping on meridian points to send stress-reduction signals to the parts of the brain that are activated by fear or negative emotions. This practice is becoming so common that you can see athletes tapping on their points during a baseball game in the dugout or before running an Olympic race to take the edge off before their performance.

Our bodies are made of energy and water. In fact, you can think of emotions as energy in motion, traveling through our meridian pathways. In traditional Eastern medicine, these pathways have been used for over 5000 years and have provided functional paths for curing disease. Recently, the meridian pathways have been proven to exist as a real anatomical system now called the Primo Vascular System (PVS).

The PVS integrates the cardiovascular, nervous, immune, and hormonal systems through the vital energy called "Qi" as an electromagnetic wave that is involved very closely with your DNA. These concepts really open the door to deeply understanding the relationship between mind, body, and the childbirth experience.

When we experience a negative event, we experience a negative emotion that disrupts the body's energy system. Many times, our brain remembers it as an implicit (subconscious) memory, and stores the information in our body ready for quick retrieval to keep us safe and prepared for the fight, flight, or freeze response when we next encounter an event we think is unsafe.

It's a great survival mechanism and comes in handy if faced by lions, tigers, and bears; however, it is not so helpful when preparing for labor with a goal of a VBAC. Also, the flood of stress hormones activated by this great protective system, if prolonged, keeps us from healing and feeling well long after childbirth itself. When I work with clients seeking the goal of having a VBAC, EFT tapping helps clear the negative emotion that was subconsciously stored in their body, and in essence clears the way so that they can be more relaxed and at peak performance level for birth.

What is Matrix Reimprinting?

Matrix Re-imprinting is a form of tapping that uses the quantum field that surrounds us to clear negative emotions and negative beliefs that are blocking us from health, wellness, trust, and even love for our bodies and the world around us. It can also be used to manifest our goals and desires.

Matrix Reimprinting evolved from EFT and was developed by EFT master Karl Dawson. Like EFT, it accesses the meridians (PVS) used in acupuncture for thousands of years.

Both EFT and Matrix Reimprinting work by bringing to mind and verbalizing, in a specific manner, an issue that you want to work with. At the same time, you tap on points on your meridians with your fingers, and this releases stress and trauma from the body's energy system, allowing the body and mind to return to a healthy physical and emotional state. Results for EFT have consistently been phenomenal, and have more far-reaching, positive results than much of our Western medical model of healing.

Conventional EFT tapping is used to take the emotional intensity out of a past memory. You are left with the ability to recall the traumatic and stressful memories without any emotional charge or stress, which is extremely useful, since negative past memories keep the body in a state of stress and can contribute to dis-ease and disease.

In Matrix Reimprinting, however, the energy of the memory is actually *transformed*. The process uses the laws of quantum physics by changing the thoughts and images we send out into the "Matrix," which is what physicist Max Planck called our energy field as early as 1944. You can go into any past memory, say and do what you wished you'd said and done, bring in new resources, and create and transform the image you have of that memory.

In Matrix Reimprinting, you see these past negative memories as images or holograms held in your energetic, or body-field. Until you transform them, you keep tuning into them on a subconscious level. They affect your health, your wellbeing, and what you attract in the present moment.

Changing the images creates both physical and emotional healing, and enables you to attract more positive experiences into your life. By tapping on the meridians of the body at the same time, the process is accelerated, because you are working directly with your vital life force energy, "Qi," which is the electromagnetic wave connected to your DNA.

Doing This on Your Own

If EFT is such an effective self-help tool that you can learn to do all by yourself, why would anyone go to a coach? Why spend the money? EFT is an amazing and effective self-help tool and it is possible to get extraordinary change with even the most basic knowledge and little or no understanding of the science and thinking behind it. However, there are times when EFT doesn't seem to work. You just get nowhere, or you may have opened up a floodgate of negative emotions and lost memories. This is where I, as an EFT coach, come in: when you are stuck, or overwhelmed.

Primarily, my role is to be a facilitator for healing work to take place and to hold a safe space for you to explore areas that your subconscious mind may not allow you to access on your own. I've helped many women and couples prepare for childbirth, especially VBACs, by shedding fear and anxiety regarding their previous birth experience.

My role is also to keep my client focused – to be a kind but firm guide of their process – to gently help them focus and resolve their issues in a supportive and comfortable environment, and keep them not just on track, but moving forward. I am a good detective; I use my language skills to creatively help them unearth their core issues and beliefs. I pose question in ways they wouldn't think of doing on their own. I believe that creative language and questioning skills are invaluable in allowing the process to flow smoothly.

It is human nature not to "go there" if "there" is too uncomfortable, either consciously or subconsciously. Some of us are masters at distraction – we've all experienced those times when cleaning, laundry, work, caring for your partner and/or children, or just hiding away in the cocoon of internet surfing or watching TV suddenly become of utmost importance and just *have* to be done. Anything to avoid the issues we know at some level we need to be working with/looking at. I know – I am quite an expert on this myself! We have all been there and done that!

As human beings, we are used to suppressing our negative thoughts and emotions. We are skilled at plowing our way through life, telling ourselves and others that everything is ok. The most common response to "How are you?" is "Fine." How often is that the truth? EFT is all about being in your truth and helping you release the negative emotions and thoughts that keep you from your end goal of love, joy, fulfillment, and an empowered VBAC.

When dealing with negative things, people often ignore what is really bothering them. But at some point, the subconscious mind will draw our attention to it in some other way, whether through physical aches and pains, depression, or anxiety or other emotional states – particularly a state of fear and doubt of being able to have a VBAC.

We might displace or project our negative feelings onto others, and this hurts our relationships. At some point the subconscious defenses leak – something happens and we are forced to confront our reality.

This is where my coaching is very helpful: to create a strategy for you to having an empowered VBAC plan, a path for you to take, and to support and guide you as necessary.

EFT is very effective for carefully resolving and changing the overall fear-tension-pain cycle of the childbirth experience. Using EFT is like becoming your own emotional detective. Can it be done on your own? Yes. But it's easier with someone to guide you, and is invaluable in allowing the process to flow smoothly and to help you unearth your core issues and beliefs.

EFT is a fast track to cognitive shifts and insights. Acknowledging these changes to ourselves can be difficult. Often, we won't notice them ourselves and it will take our family, friends or colleagues to point them out. I help my clients bring these shifts into conscious awareness as they happen.

That is how I see my role: supporting you to move along your chosen track of wanting a VBAC to happen, being a clear channel for labor to happen gracefully – being aware when you head off track and pulling you gently back, looking for those patterns, helping you examine these patterns, and gain new insights and perspectives.

Childbirth with Grace Tapping Points

These are the locations and names of the tapping points for EFT and Matrix Reimprinting that I use with my clients.

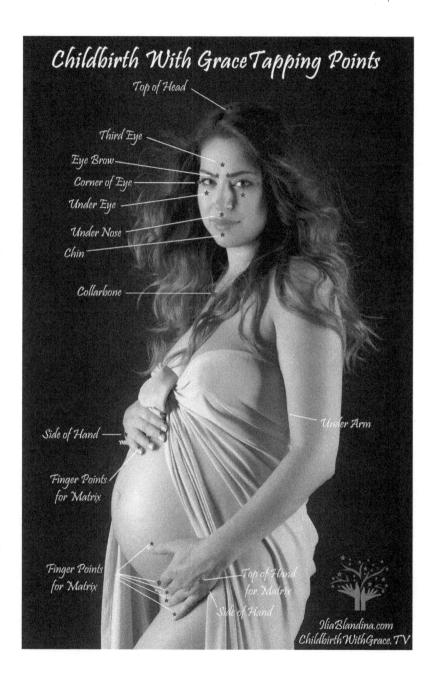

How to Tap

So this is how we do EFT (tapping). Refer to the previous photo for a visual location of all the points. The pace of tapping on the points should be at a moderate cadence. And you want to do this with enough pressure that you feel it but not so hard that you feel pain; imagine tapping your fingers on a table. Sometimes you will be using two fingers, sometimes four, depending on the location and size of the meridian point.

Location and Order of Tapping Points

Side of Hand Point: We always begin with the side of the hand point. The side of the hand point is located between the base of the pinky and the top of the wrist, in the fleshy part of your hand where, if you were practicing karate, you would be chopping a board of wood.

You will be tapping the side of your hand by using your non-dominant hand. If you are right handed, for example, you will take the four fingers of your right hand and tap on the side of your left hand over and over again.

Top of Head Point: The next point is the very top of the head, also called your crown. Because it is a very large area, use four fingers. It's okay to use the fingers of either hand.

Third Eye Point: Many practitioners don't use this point, but I have found it to be very helpful. If you were to draw a line connecting your eyebrows and go about an inch above, that is where you want to be. It happens to be a major trauma point in the meridian system. Use your index and middle finger of either hand to tap right on that spot.

Eyebrow Point: This is close to the bridge of the nose, right where the eyebrow starts. You can tap on your right eyebrow, your left eyebrow, or both at the same time with both hands. It doesn't matter.

Corner of Eye Point: You want to go between the outer ridge of the eye socket and the temple. Don't tap on the temple or too close to your eye. Again, you are you use your index and middle fingers of one hand to tap there. You can also tap on both sides simultaneously if you would like.

Under Eye Point: This is located one inch below the center of the pupil (when looking straight forward), on the bone. Using the index and middle fingers again, you can also tap on the right or left side or both sides simultaneously.

Under Nose Point: This point is between the bottom of the nose and the top of the upper lip. Use your index and middle fingers to tap.

Chin Point: This point is actually just below your bottom lip, on the crease that you have above your chin. Use the same two fingers, index and middle, to tap there.

Collar Bone Point: The collar bone is where a man would tie his neck tie knot. Touch each side of your collar bone with the fingers of either open hand. Touch one side with your thumb, and the other with your middle finger. Now move your hand just slightly below the bones, and tap there as if patting yourself on the chest with your fingertips.

Under Arm Point: This point is located four fingers below the armpit on each side of the body. For a woman, it is where your bra strap generally crosses over. This is a large area, so again, use all four fingers of your dominant hand and tap the opposite side of your body. So if you are tapping with your right hand, you would tap under your left arm four inches under your armpit.

Those are all the points I use for EFT. The additional points used for Matrix Re-imprinting are located on the fingertips, as shown in the picture. I will go over how to use them later in the book.

The Set-up Phrase and Reminder Statements

When tapping, many people get stuck on what to say. But there is actually a formula of how to structure your thoughts. The first place we tap is at the side of the hand and what we will say is known as the set-up phrase.

The **set-up phrase** is the first portion of EFT, a statement you make and repeat out loud while you tap on the side of the hand. It goes like this: **"Even though I feel** [blank] **about** [blank]**, I deeply and completely accept myself."** You say this statement three times.

1. "Even though I feel [blank] about [blank], I deeply and completely accept myself."
2. "Even though I feel [blank] about [blank], I deeply and completely accept myself."
3. "Even though I feel [blank] about [blank], I deeply and completely accept myself."

What goes in the **[blank]** is where people get stuck. The most effective way to use EFT is by filling in those blanks about **what you feel** about a particular issue **and where** it shows up **in your body.**

It's more important for you to **focus on specific events** than on general or global statements. The majority of self-help videos out there are too general. The best way to use EFT is to be as specific as possible. And the best way to use EFT on a physical condition is to work on the emotional aspects of the condition.

For example, you could say, "Even though I feel *aggravated when I look in the mirror and I see that I have a C-section scar on my belly,* I deeply and completely accept myself."

Now when you think about that statement, do you feel something in your body? Is there a tension, tightness, a constriction, an ache, pain anywhere in your body? If there is, go ahead and include it because it will make the statement even more specific:

"Even though I feel *aggravated when I look in the mirror and I see that I have a C-section scar on my belly,* and I feel the aggravation as *tightness in my shoulders,* I deeply and completely accept myself."

Before you start tapping – but once you know the specific event and the emotion you are dealing with – you want to ask yourself, "How intensely do I feel about this issue?" Are you feeling really intense, moderately intense, or not so intense? This helps to track your progress.

The traditional way to do this is by giving the emotion a number from 0 to 10. Zero means you have no intensity, 5 you are moderately intense and 10 is very high intensity. This is also called **Subjective Units of Distress (SUDs)**. Of course, if it is zero, you don't have to tap on it, so generally you want to come up with an event that has a SUDs level of 5 or more.

Identify your SUDs level before starting to tap, then say the set-up statement three times while tapping on the side of your hand as previously described:

1. "Even though I feel aggravated when I look in the mirror and I see that I have a C-section scar on my belly, and I feel the aggravation as tightness in my shoulders, I deeply and completely accept myself."
2. "Even though I feel aggravated when I look in the mirror and I see that I have a C-section scar on my belly, and I feel the aggravation as tightness in my shoulders, I deeply and completely accept myself."
3. "Even though I feel aggravated when I look in the mirror and I see that I have a C-section scar on my belly, and I feel the aggravation as tightness in my shoulders, I deeply and completely accept myself."

After that, you go to the remaining points from the top of the head to under the arm, saying *"This aggravation and tightness in my shoulders."* In other words, the formula is to say the word "this" in front of the emotion and sensation in your body you've identified in your set-up statement.

It doesn't matter how many times you say it at each point. Start at the top of the head and keep repeating the **reminder statement** at all the points in the following order:

Top of Head: "This aggravation and tightness in my shoulders."
Third Eye: "This aggravation and tightness in my shoulders."
Eyebrow: "This aggravation and tightness in my shoulders."
Corner of Eye: "This aggravation and tightness in my shoulders."
Under Eye: "This aggravation and tightness in my shoulders."
Under Nose: "This aggravation and tightness in my shoulders."
Chin: "This aggravation and tightness in my shoulders."
Collar Bone: "This aggravation and tightness in my shoulders."
Under Arm: "This aggravation and tightness in my shoulders."

Shifting Aspects

The next thing you need to be aware of is recognizing shifting aspects. So it will come in handy if you have an EFT journal and pen by your side when you are tapping on your own. **Shifting aspects** are when another thought, event, sensation, or emotion comes up while you are tapping on the original specific event and the emotion and sensation you gave a SUD measurement to.

Shifting aspects happen because our neural pathways recognize, categorize, generalize, and put things into the areas of our brain where they make sense to us. This makes everything connected to everything else – especially within a belief, an issue, or a specific event.

So, what happens is that during a tapping round, another thought floats in. This is where you can easily get fooled into thinking the techniques are not working. It's not that EFT doesn't work, it's just that another aspect of the problem showed up and you did not recognize the shift. An example of this would be if your thoughts started to drift away from feeling aggravation towards remembering the look given to you when your practitioner came in the room to tell you about needing to do a C-section.

The most important thing you can do when working on your own is to *not follow the shift.* Do not go there midstream while you are still tapping on one specific event. Instead, write it down and get back to it later. In our example, stay with the aggravation of seeing your C-section scar on your belly, because otherwise you can get way far off topic and not resolve the triggers from the specific issue you are working on.

You can work on what came up later, write it down in your journal and let it go for now. This prevents you from feeling overwhelmed due to jumping around from issue to issue. It will also prevent you from giving up because you suddenly think there are too many pieces to the puzzle.

Testing Your Tapping

The idea is to continue tapping on a specific problem until the intensity of the emotion goes down. It may take a couple of rounds of tapping. With each round of tapping, you should re-evaluate your SUDs rate. Continue until it is a zero.

If your SUDs do not get to a zero, then you may be experiencing a shifting aspect – so pay close attention to what comes up in your thoughts while you are tapping and write them down. Another reason why you may not have a lower SUDs rate is due to dehydration. Remember, emotions are energy in motion through the Primo Vascular System (meridians), and if you are low in fluids, it will be harder to tap the emotions through. Being pregnant alone requires more hydration needs, so always have water on hand and take a few sips after each tapping round.

Wait, There Is More!

In the next chapter, I will be talking about how to use EFT in the heat of the moment during labor. Using EFT in labor is much easier in one sense, but more difficult in another.

It is easier if you have done EFT before labor to clear up all the fears and doubts you have about trusting your body to have a VBAC *before* feeling any contractions. During labor, for the most part, you don't have to come up with a specific event to focus on for EFT to be effective. Being in the moment of labor is specific enough.

By the same token, doing EFT only in labor can be harder because you have not cleared your negative emotions of fear and doubt from past events. What happens is your subconscious mind has collected negative aspects of previous events in order to keep you safe. If you don't do the work before labor, tapping only during labor may not be enough to quiet your internal monologue that will run through your mind in the height of the labor process.

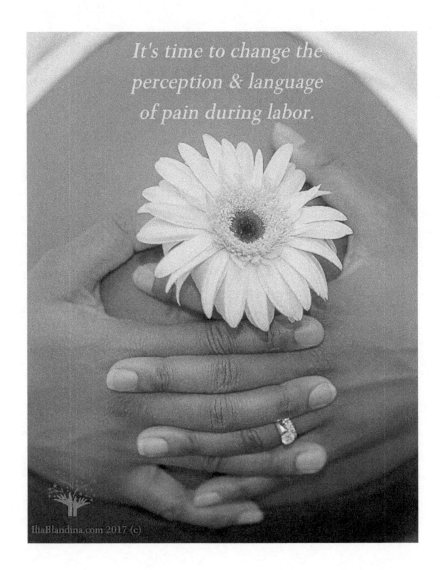

It's time to change the perception & language of pain during labor.

IliaBlandina.com 2017 (c)

CHAPTER 8

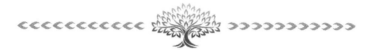

Changing Your Perception of Pain

"Perception is reality, and I hallucinate."

~ GARY BLANDINA

The Dilemma of Change

There are so many ways to approach the subject of pain during labor. The best way is your own way. But how can you know how to deal with it if you have no reference point? Even one birth to the next can be completely different. It can also change from one contraction to the next.

Your first baby was a C-section; maybe you never even experienced labor. Maybe your C-section was because the baby was breech. What does labor feel like? There lies the mystery; even if you know what labor feels like the next birth can be completely different!

So, you may be asking yourself, "How can I possibly prepare when I can't really anticipate what it will be like?" Fear sets in; you freeze and start to rethink the whole idea of a VBAC. Wait! Before you wave that white flag of surrender, let me help you change your perception of pain during labor and therefore change your reality. Yes, we can do this together, way before the first contraction comes.

Change Your Perception Ceremony

First and foremost, we must change the words we use. From now on, we will call your sensations during labor *contractions,* and we will release the word *pain* to spirit. Better yet, we can also call the sensations *rushes, surges,* or *waves.* Now would be a good time to have a small fire ceremony outside. Write the words *"Labor Pain"* on a small piece of paper; go outside and set fire to those words in a safe container while holding the intention of releasing the association of labor and giving birth with pain.

When I work with clients and help them plan this intention ceremony, it opens their mind to a new way of thinking about labor. I guide them to consider the best phase of the moon to do this. It will all depend on what you are trying to work on: release, contemplation, rebirth, fresh starts, manifestation, gravidity, clarity, or fullness of power. You can get this information from the VBAC Tool Kit, which will help you decide when best to do it.

Breathe, You Can Do This

The second step that I help my clients learn is the importance of being aware of their breath. Oh, I know what you are thinking: "Okay, here we go another Lamaze book...." Nope, you couldn't be further from the truth. Hang in there with me; you'll see where I go with this. Even though it may seem obvious, there's more to this than meets the eye. Remember, "Perception is reality."

There is an old saying: *"Live one day at a time."* In labor, one day can be the longest day of your life. I used to advise my clients to just concentrate on one contraction at a time. **Now it's time to go deeper! We need to take it to** *"one breath at a time!"*

Your breathing is already perfect. You don't have to memorize how to breathe or at what cadence you should be breathing. Throw out that Lamaze book; you're not going to remember all of that in the heat of the moment anyway. You're not going to forget how to breathe. **Instead, I teach my clients to be** *aware* **of how they are breathing.**

Labor contractions are never static or motionless. They change in location and intensity moment by moment. Contractions come and go, taking the form of rushes, surges, and waves. But your memory of and beliefs and emotions about the sensations you feel with the contractions can become fixed in your mind.

If a negative memory comes up while experiencing labor contractions, it may dictate how you experience the present moment and can affect how you breathe. When working with my clients, I remind them that breath awareness helps keep their uterus and the baby well-oxygenated. A smooth flow of oxygen to the uterine muscle will help the contractions be more effective, lessen the work load for the muscle fibers (which means less pain), and maintain oxygen flow to the baby via the placenta.

This would be a good time to mention that I also give my clients a nutritional formula for preventing iron deficiency anemia. Remember, your red blood cells carry oxygen through your body. Because your blood volume plasma increases 50% by the time you are 12 weeks pregnant, you are likely to be one of many pregnant women prone to anemia just by the dilution effect alone.

With all that being said, this is why I always say that it's not about planning, it's about clearing the way. The exercises that I have taught my clients not only help develop the skills to deal with contractions, but they also can help access specific memories that have negative emotions such as fear, self-doubt, shame, embarrassment, anger, and beliefs of not being in a safe world.

These negative emotions, if not cleared prior to labor, can actually intensify the pain you feel during a contraction, which leads you into the fear-tension-pain cycle. If you get caught in that cycle, it will cause your present experience of the birth process to spiral out of control in your mind. And, unfortunately, it will lead to suffering and struggle during labor.

With breath awareness, the idea is to let go and just notice what is happening. It is not about affirmations. Instead it is about training your mind to have pure awareness of your breath while tapping on your meridian points (as explained in the previous chapter).

Here's how it worked out for one of my clients. After working with her on all the negative things she remembered from her previous birth, I taught her how to elicit a simulated contraction sensation using ice. Yes, you can really practice these techniques before you ever feel your first labor contraction. It's safe and easy to simulate labor using ice!

Ice Cube Exercise
- Mild pain: Hold in hand (both hands if partner taps on you)
- Moderate pain: Hold on wrist (both wrists if partner taps on you)
- Severe pain: Hold behind ear (both ears if partner taps on you)

I had learned this technique during my last pregnancy and have taught it to all of my clients. They have found it to be a very helpful way to learn how they will respond to mild, moderate, and severe sensations.

Back to my client, Lisa. She so wanted to not freak out during the contractions. Her first baby was a C-section because of breech presentation. She didn't know what a contraction felt like, because the C-section was planned. She was committed to having a trial of labor after C-section (TOLAC), but after helping her resolve all her regrets from the first birth, we had to prepare for the real thing.

I taught her how to use ice on specific points on her body that would simulate initial, mild contractions. I also taught her how to do this exercise with her partner. I taught her how to apply the ice and where. Next, I instructed her to be in the part of her home where she most wanted to labor.

Lisa was planning to stay in her bathtub for as long as possible, so most of the time that was where she and her partner did the exercises. Her partner was responsible for timing the application of the ice and holding the ice. Lisa just had to be aware of her breath and tap on her meridian points. No words had to be used.

As she got the hang of this, I taught her how to intensify the simulation by applying ice to different points on her body. I also taught her other techniques that can be combined with tapping and breath awareness. The idea behind learning different ways to change your perception is that you don't know which one will work for you during real labor. Both she and her partner became proficient at all the techniques.

The best part of all this was what surfaced during her training exercises. She started having memories of when she felt insecure in the past. Part of my coaching was to have her write down what came up during the ice exercises so that we could work on the specific events and beliefs that may cause her to lose confidence in herself or her body and give up her goal to have a VBAC. I was able to teach her to perceive her contraction sensations from a different, more positive perspective. Yes, she went on to have a successful vaginal birth after C-section!

*****

Precision Total Awareness Exercise

Another layer that can be applied to being aware of your breath is called non-focused awareness, a concentration technique practiced by Samurai warriors that you can apply to labor.

By mastering this technique, you will become less self-centered and self-conscious, because you will be able to incorporate everything around you as part of your labor experience and not simply hyper-focus on contractions. Non-focused awareness helps you to learn how to use all your senses to control your perception and therefore your reality.

Swordsmen practice non-focused awareness of the total moment. Of course, their motivation was that at any moment, a lapse of concentration could get them killed! At least you don't have to worry about that. The idea is to keep yourself from having an internal mental struggle that is triggered by your external environment. Samurai concentration is fierce; they are totally present, aware of everything but not distracted by anything.

Developing a warrior goddess outlook in labor is one of the best ways to cope with fear, exhaustion, and pain. This will keep you focused on the immediate situation in its wholeness, rather than letting any isolated fragment grab your attention. When you practice, and incorporate staying open to all sensations, moment-to-moment, pain is removed from its central place in your awareness and it just becomes a contraction, surge, rush, or wave of sensation.

This technique was extremely important for my client Emily. She was looking forward to her labor, but not sure how she would feel being naked in front of strangers as well as the family and friends that she really wanted to be present during the birth.

During labor, everything around you become a part of your birth experience. During her work with me, Emily was able to release her fears and negative beliefs about exposing her body during labor, her VBAC was successful, and she was incredibly glad her family and friends were there to witness the miracle of birth.

Non-Focused Awareness means staying open to all of your senses while at the same time tapping on your meridian points. You'll notice, below, that I do not include the underarm point during labor because you may have discomfort or difficulty reaching that area when you are having contractions. Here is how it works: In this exercise, you will alternate from softening one of your senses while tapping on a point and then saying softly out loud what that sense has noticed. In other words, alternating between physical action and spoken word focused observation.

- **Tap on your head.** You soften your sight.
- **Tap on your third eye and eye brow.** Say out loud softly, *"I see the sheets."*
- **Tap on the corner of your eyes.** You soften what you hear.
- **Tap under your eyes.** Say out loud softly, *"I hear the clock."*
- **Tap under your nose.** You soften your sense of smell.
- **Tap on your chin point.** Say out loud softly, *"I smell coffee or food."*
- **Tap on your collar bone point.** You soften the sensations on your skin.
- **Tap on your head.** Say out loud softly, *"I feel my partner's touch."*
- **Tap on your third eye and eye brow.** Your taste buds soften while you eat your popsicle.
- **Tap on the corner of your eyes.** Say out loud softly, *"I taste my orange popsicle."*
- **Tap under your eyes.** Your intuition softly comes to your attention.

- **Tap under your nose.** You let others know by saying out loud softly, *"I need to change position."*
- **Tap on your chin point.** As labor progresses you allow yourself to become softly aware of body sensation.
- **Tap on your collar bone point.** You let your partner know, *"I feel pressure or stretching."*

Non-focused awareness is practiced by shifting between non-verbal and verbal awareness. This allows you to let your needs and sensation be known as well as controlling your internal monologue. You will be able to prevent your internal monologue from going rogue on you and veering into negative awareness mode.

By practicing this technique before labor, you can uncover any tendencies you may have toward a rogue negative internal monologue. When I work with my clients, I have them write down these rogue thoughts no matter how strange and unconnected they may seem at the time. With my coaching, they are able to uncover the hidden meaning or belief that may hinder progress towards their goal of a VBAC.

Remember, the majority of the time it is fear and the stress hormones that are released that can stop labor. The goal is to decrease the stress hormones of cortisol and adrenaline. By practicing how to control your perception in labor, you can naturally let go and release your own oxytocin, which is the hormone of love. **Here is the big secret, love and fear cannot coexist!**

When you are shifting from non-verbal to verbal non-focused awareness, silently say what you are noticing to yourself, and then say it out loud. Your partner can also give you cues. Ask your partner to practice speaking slowly, allowing time for you to listen through a full breath or two.

If any distractions occur during your tapping exercise, you or your partner may include it in the cue, for example, the sound of an airplane flying overhead, or the sound of the phone ringing or door slamming shut accidently (the sound of the clock was used in the example above). Gently being aware of your environment will keep the awareness broad and non-focused.

*****

The Wave Tapping Sequence

Here is how you combine awareness of breath, tapping, and non-focused awareness. I call it the Wave Tapping Sequence. When tapping on the third eye point and eye brow point, do it simultaneously by using your fingers of one hand in a claw position. Your thumb at one eye brow point, the index and middle finger on the third eye, and your ring finger at the opposite eye brow point.

First bring your attention to your breath while either you or your partner tap on your meridian points as follows:

- **Tap on your head.** Become aware of your breath. Inhale and exhale using the diaphragm.
- **Tap on your third eye and eye brow.** Listen to the sounds you hear within.
- **Tap on the corner of your eyes.** Listen to the sounds just outside your ears.
- **Tap under your eyes.** Listen to the sounds at the edge of your room.
- **Tap under your nose.** Listen to the sounds from the next room.
- **Tap on your chin point.** Listen to the sounds outside the building.
- **Tap on your collar bone point.** Listen to the sounds down the street.

- **Tap on your head.** Now bring your attention to your breath. Inhale and exhale.
- **Tap on your third eye and eyebrow points.** Listen to the sounds down the street.
- **Tap on the corner of your eyes.** Listen to the sounds outside the building.
- **Tap under your eyes.** Listen to the sounds from the next room.
- **Tap under your nose.** Listen to the sounds at the edge of your room.
- **Tap on your chin point.** Listen to sounds just outside your ears.
- **Tap on your collar bone.** Listen to the sounds within.
- **Tap on your head.** Become aware of your breath. Inhale and exhale using the diaphragm.

Notice how you controlled your awareness from inside out, then outside in. Again, the underarm point was skipped because it may be uncomfortable to reach. This pattern can be repeated again and again.

Although the Wave Tapping Sequence is designed to be a loop pattern, it is a good idea to not expect to use one technique continuously through labor. Your mind will not be able to concentrate intensely on one thing for long periods of time when you are in active labor. You may find yourself floating through different techniques.

With practice, you become more flexible. You will flow from one technique to another without labeling. The key is always being aware of your breath. If you are in a quiet room, non-focused awareness may be more difficult to use. This is when listening to music or sounds of nature may come in handy, so start making your labor music playlist.

When the mind is focused, breathing becomes slow and rhythmical. Steady breathing calms the sympathetic nervous system and allows for better focus and optimal body functions. This technique prevents you from hyperventilating or holding your breath. On the other hand, if you find yourself holding your breath and bearing down, it may be time to push, so remember to let your helper know when you start feeling these sensations.

*****

If non-focused awareness doesn't seem to be working, consider:

- Are you looking around too actively? Keep your gaze soft and only on what is in front of you – or maybe it's time to walk around or move your hips from side to side.
- Are you judging or being analytical? Concentrate on your senses and let go of judging thoughts. If they pop in, let them pop out.
- Are you easily distracted, losing your train of thought? Have someone give you cues. (Make cue cards).
- Is your personal awareness moving too fast or too slow? Change your pace. Sometimes you have to go faster during the more intense contractions; this will help you from thinking too much or worrying. You can also try slowing down by using the Wave Tapping Sequence.

This is why practicing with your partner is so important, because you have another person who knows your non-verbal cues well and can help you switch up techniques.

How to Use These Techniques with Your Partner

Partners can use non-focused awareness as well. Anticipating the birth of a child can be pretty exciting, but also becomes boring after a while. It's a "hurry up and wait" scenario that can be both physically and mentally exhausting. Remember, labor is similar to a marathon: you don't want to use all your energy in the first few miles. If your partner practices non-focused awareness during labor, they will be more aware of your needs and will feel more present and calm at the time of the baby's birth.

When I help, my clients become proficient with these exercises from a place of love and then they practice with their partner, it helps them prepare to work together during labor. Partners learn to start using cues as soon as the contraction begins and deliver the cue during the inhale, so that you will know what to focus on during the exhale. Use the same imagery during a series of contractions.

Repetition is soothing and will guide you to master your concentration. Too much creative variety can become frustrating. It's best to practice before labor to discover which phrase, imagery, or adjective works best for you.

When I say it's not about planning, it's about clearing the way to your best possible birth journey, I mean that the big shift that needs to happen is in your perception and your internal monologue. Without these techniques, your monologue can easily slip into this: "Oh no! Another contraction! I don't want to do this anymore! I can't do this! Stop that beeping! Stop talking! Shut the door! This is taking too long! I can't! I give up! I want a C-section!" I've seen it happen all too often.

Can you practice these techniques on your own? Absolutely! I encourage you to set aside a time to practice every day, on your own and with your partner. This is important because how you then respond to your real contractions will become automatic and empowered. Also, your partner will start learning your non-verbal cues, and it will be easier for them to pick up on these cues when you are in labor.

If, as you practice, you get stuck along the way, you can always reach out and contact me to see if personalized coaching makes sense for you. Either way, the idea is to transform your internal monologue to: "I notice my belly tightening. I hear my breath. I hear people talking. I hear my breath. I hear a beep. I hear my breath." Alternating between hearing your breath and what you hear in the environment while tapping on your meridian points.

Other techniques include ways to help change your perception of the contractions by focusing on different parts of the contraction itself. For example, the edge of the discomfort, the edge of your comfort, softening the awareness of your discomfort, and focusing on the center of your discomfort.

All of these techniques have helped my clients make friends with their contractions, rushes, surges, waves, and pressure. The idea is to learn and practice how to use your curiosity to closely examine and yet be open to all the sensations in your body while you are in labor.

Your partner can also help you soften around the contraction with the use of cues. The more you resist something, the more it persists. By the same token, what you embrace dissolves. The overall goal is to help you get into a mental space where you are embracing your birth journey just as you would hold your baby after the birth.

Stopping the Fear-Tension-Pain Cycle

By learning to say yes to your contractions, you will find the inner peace needed during labor. Exploring the sensations you have during contractions is a method of making friends with them. By getting to know your contraction, the tension and fear created by resisting it goes away. Decreasing tension and fear leads to changing your perception of pain! The Fear-Tension-Pain cycle stops!

You become curious about the contraction instead of pushing it away or trying to distract yourself. Remember, your contraction sensation is always changing. The problem is that our memory of the pain becomes embedded in our mind, especially when we attach a strong emotion to it, like fear.

When we memorize the sensation, location, and the meaning we assign to it, we then begin responding to the history of the pain rather than what is happening in the present moment. This makes our response to the contraction get stuck in pain mode.

Ongoing intense pain is exhausting and overwhelms your mind. Eventually you start to think it is unmanageable, and the pain begins to define your whole being. It takes courage to embrace the contractions and let go of the pain by looking at every contraction separately from where each begins and ends. In between contractions, bring your attention to your breath. Inhale love, and release any tension with an exhale.

Another way to approach this is to become aware of the parts of your body that are comfortable. Remember that scene in *Raiders of the Lost Ark* when Indiana Jones points out what areas can be kissed because that is where he is not feeling any pain from being dragged behind the truck?

Where is your body soft and relaxed? Maybe your partner can also kiss those areas too. Again, always begin with the awareness of your breath. With each breath, bring full attention to where your body is not hurting. This is a very powerful technique because it will help your body release oxytocin and endorphins as we discussed in Chapter 6.

There are many variations of these techniques. The key is to practice them and become aware of any negative thoughts or emotions that may come up. This is how you will be able to identify any fear-based thinking. Start a tapping journal and use basic EFT to bring down the emotional intensity of specific events you remember that are connected to the negative emotions. When you get rid of the fear, the tension in your body is released and the pain goes away.

Once the negative emotions are gone, go back to practicing the tapping sequences with the use of ice to simulate labor. I encourage you to practice on your own *and* with your birth partner so you are totally prepared, just in case your labor starts when you are alone.

If you find it difficult to do it on your own, you can always reach out to me to set up a phone chat. When my clients practice with me, they are able to clear the negative emotions that are keeping them blocked; they are better able to practice with their partner without engaging in a negative internal monologue that will prevent their labor from progressing. Always be mindful of what emotions are triggered while you practice, write them down, and tap to neutralize them before the big event.

Remember the goal is to be as clear and present during your labor as possible. This will help you emanate love and empowered strength. In doing so, you will get that reflected back to you by your practitioners. We are wired to reflect back what we see. So, if you present yourself with fear, your practitioners will also be fearful for you, and that usually leads to too much intervention and eventually a C-section.

Mystic Awareness Techniques

The Center of Your Contraction

These techniques help you focus on the unseen part of labor. First, focus on the center of your contraction, and as you do this, notice that the center is not fixed. It may move in very subtle ways, sometimes with a rhythm, and the movement may be slow or fast. When observing the center of your contraction, consider the stillness of the eye of a hurricane.

The "eye" of the hurricane relates to the pervasive Oriental celestial symbol of the "hole," which is represented in the disc of a Chinese Jade pendant. This is also called Pi, representing heaven. It represents the concept of the zenith of stillness, a void through which one may pass out of the world of space and time into spacelessness and timelessness. It therefore has a close relationship with the concepts of time and space and the mystic center where there is no time or space, the mystic "nothingness". This is why, by concentrating on the center of your contraction, you are better able to find the absence of pain.

Despite the symbol of a hurricane as being a destructive force, it is also symbolic of a cleansing effect by clearing everything that might get in the way, and thereby provides a clean, new beginning. While you practice these techniques, consider what needs to be cleared away in order to welcome your new life into the world of the earth plane.

What is your storm of worry that fills your mind from time to time? Pay attention to your inner monologue. Write down what comes up. What are the fears that keep you up at night? What triggers your fear, anger, sadness, regret, shame?

As always, use awareness of your breath to become centered. When considering the analogy of the eye of a hurricane, be aware that the breath and a hurricane have the Element of Air. This will guide you to the state of being, the state of creation, transformation, and restoration.

The Air's spiritual quality is always identified as the pure essence of "being," itself. Though the air may move or become altered due to the terrain it moves over, it is always there, neither being born nor dying, only appearing in different forms.

You may also find the center moves in rhythm with your breath. If the sensation increases as you breathe in, imagine moving deeper into the center as you exhale. With each breath, notice how both the center and the sensation are in constant movement. You can also focus your Third Eye on the center and tap on that.

Your Contraction as a Spiral

Let's focus on your contraction as a spiral. Why is the spiral such a compelling shape? Why does it have a positive meaning for every culture? Could it be because we, on this tiny planet, live in a spiral galaxy? The spiral is the oldest symbol known to be used in spiritual practices.

Although its meaning varies depending on the culture, it can be found in the artwork of most people of Europe, Asia, Africa, and the Americas. Consider this: the oldest spiral symbols can be seen in Ireland at the megalithic site of Newgrange, where these mysterious symbols date back to about 3,200 B.C. Focusing your awareness of your contraction as a spiral will help you connect with many ancestors that gave birth before you and helped bring you to this point.

The spiral imagery in your contraction reflects the universal pattern of growth and evolution and represents the goddess, the womb, fertility, and life force energy.

Reflected in the natural world, the spiral is found in human physiology, plants, minerals, animals, energy patterns, weather, growth, and death. When one looks at these symbols from a spiritual context, one finds they have profound meaning and depth as symbols of unity and ascension. It is a sacred symbol that reminds us of our evolving journey in life.

Spirals also represent movement through experiences in life. View the spiral as the symbol of one's progressive development, growth, and expansion as you make your journey towards the center and towards the light. At the spiral's center is where you find spiritual balance and realize your deep connection to the eternal forces of nature and the universe.

As you move into the spiral of your contraction, you are letting go of undesired aspects of your ego, possessions, and worry about other people's perceptions of you and moving towards your core self. You will gain insights into your personal beliefs and behaviors on this inward journey and move into higher conscious awareness.

As you move back out, you are growing and connecting to Source Energy of All That IS in a loving, harmonious, and collaborative way. Yes, you are in collaboration with your body, contraction, and baby.

The path of life resembles a spiral. We seem to pass the same point over and over again, but from a different perspective each time. If you flatten the spiral and look forward or back at yourself, it is like the onion. Visualize metaphysically peeling off more of the onion each time we pass the same issue in the spiral of our life and labor.

This technique may uncover many layers of fear and doubt that you weren't aware of. Use your journal to write your thoughts or memories of specific events and negative emotions down. Review EFT in Chapter 7 and use it to neutralize any negative feelings. This helps you to peel the onion so that you don't come back to the same issue of fear and doubt. You will become empowered and can move into higher energy vibration more quickly before and during labor.

When used as a personal talisman, the spiral helps consciousness to accept the turnings and changes of life and the birth process as it evolves.

I used these techniques with my client, Amy. She had been at 8 centimeters for three hours and was on the verge of getting a C-section. Luckily, her doctor was open to alternative methods and was willing to give her more time. I had just come on duty and he said, "Can you work your magic?" I jumped in and, after assessing Amy, determined that her baby was in a posterior position, meaning the back of the head was against her tail bone – and that is the hardest way for the baby to maneuver through the birth canal.

She had a doula, and they had tried many positions to encourage the baby to turn and get in better alignment with her pelvis. I asked Amy if she could go back to her hands and knees one more time. I tapped on her meridian points while guiding her to breathe and imagine her contraction as a spiral, moving back and forth from the center out to the edges and back into the center.

I helped her become aware of her breath. Ultimately, I helped her to use her contraction spiral to open and expand her cervix and rotate the baby. Voila! Within 15 minutes, it was time to push!

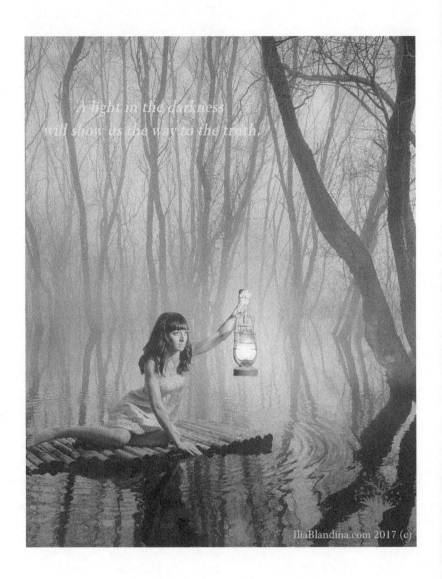

A light in the darkness
will show us the way to the truth.

CHAPTER 9

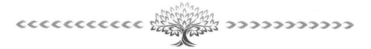

The Uphill Climb

"If we hope to create a non-violent world
where respect and kindness replace fear and hatred...
we must begin with how we treat each other at the beginning of life.
For that is where our deepest patterns are set
From these roots grow fear and alienation... or love and trust."

~ SUZANNE ARMS

The Difference between US and Them

Midwives attend over 70% of the births in Europe and Japan, yet in the United States they attend less than 8%. Of the developed world, the United States has the second worst newborn death rate and one of the highest maternal mortality rates among all industrialized countries.

This is the outcome when you are a century or more past midwives attending the majority of births. We are losing a lot of knowledge because when births went into the hospital in this country, the midwives were not allowed to follow it there.

Today, we must rediscover how easy birth can be when we don't try to make it complicated by insisting on interventions that in most cases are not needed. Ideally, births should be attended only by an experienced, motherly, and low-profile midwife.

The modeling of this should be included in the education of medical students. The fact that very few doctors have observed a normal birth is sad. In many medical circles, there are some people who claim that in the future, most women will prefer to have an elective C-section.

Women who understand the importance of the birth process and journey cannot accept that C-section is the future of birth. The majority of women have an intuitive knowledge of the importance of what is happening when a baby is born. Because of this, we as women need to reestablish our autonomy concerning birth.

Media Perpetuating Fear of Birth

Women have been made afraid of birth because they do not have an image of what birth looks like. American women watch TV shows like *A Baby Story* or *Maternity Ward*, and true to style, the media edits out the "boring" parts and includes only the scary and dramatic things that can happen in order to maintain ratings up.

So instead of showing birth as being a calm, peaceful, state of bliss, these shows instill a lot of fear in women around birth. Every birth you see on these shows are women screaming and being rushed down the hallway and looking like an absolute dire emergency is happening. These shows are passing on that these dramatic and scary birth stories are what should be expected as the norm.

It's no wonder the average woman doesn't feel confident about giving birth. The whole culture is telling them birth is a scary and dangerous thing, and more than likely something will go wrong, so you better give birth in a hospital or else you run the risk of a bad outcome!

All of these drives women to expect to have a traumatic experience, so they figure they might as well have the baby in the hospital and take advantage of getting an epidural. Women are literally terrified into thinking they should start with interventions instead of trusting their bodies to know how to give birth.

Each of these shows set up the birth to be dramatic, extremely frightening and there is always some sort of danger that sets up the doctor to come in and save the day, like the knight in shining armor. Obviously, if the doctor is playing the "I think your baby is in danger card," the dream of having a normal vaginal birth is over.

Unfortunately, this is one of the greatest manipulative techniques ever. When a woman starts to question, "Wait, why do we need to do this?" "Is there something else we can do?" the first thing the doctor will say is, "Oh, it's for the good of the baby." Whether it is or not, you'll do anything, because if you go on to question it, well, now you are a bad mom.

This has been such a problem that I actually have written a prescription for my clients that said, "Do not watch medical shows on TV or the internet. It is contraindicated during pregnancy or the childbearing years." Then I would give them a prescription to watch comedies and make love.

Barriers of Vaginal Birth

Another battle centers around time: delivery has to happen within certain time constraints or else. Women end up getting only one side of the story, and then it becomes easy to convince them to have one procedure or another, especially because there is a huge power disparity. When the doctor tells a woman in labor, "I think we need to do x," the doctor may think he is offering the woman an option, but what the woman hears is the expert is advising her to take one clear and true course.

As we all know, the C-section rate is climbing in this country. Why? What is really underneath this? First, C-sections are extremely doctor-friendly. Instead of having to wait for a woman to go into labor and laboring for an average of 20 hours for first-time moms and approximately 12 hours for second-time moms, a doctor can just schedule a C-section. This avoids having to be available at any time during the day or night, seven days a week. C-sections are a 20- to 45-minute surgery and then "I'll be home for dinner."

In fact, in my career I've seen doctors boast about how fast they can do a C-section, I've heard about and seen records as fast as 12 minutes from start to finish. I'm not kidding; all you have to do is look at the surgical records. The time of entering the operating room (OR) suite, first incision, final closure of abdomen and time leaving the OR suite is always recorded.

There was a study that showed C-section rates over a 24-hour period, and what it revealed was that the peaks in C-sections were at 4 pm and 10 pm. So, it's very obvious that at 4 in the afternoon, it's because it's the end of a long day and the doctor needs to get home. The 10 pm C-sections are about "I don't want to be up all night."

Some doctors even take advantage of a client's interest in a C-section by offering it as an option over having a vaginal birth. It certainly makes the life of an obstetrician much less complicated that way.

The bottom line is that obstetricians are trained surgeons, so their focus is to look for and be on alert for the worst-case scenario. *They were not taught to see birth as a normal event.* Their perspective is biased to look for and always predict for the worst-case scenario and how to avoid it.

The second underlying problem is the risk of litigation. Many doctors are trained by their mentors that *"they can never fault you if you just section them, so when in doubt, just section them."* This mentality brings to the forefront that the standard at the end of the day is that if you do the C-section, you did everything you could to get the baby out and the C-section becomes a faster go-to intervention instead of letting the woman have enough time to go at her own pace.

So, the current thinking is if we might get sued, it's better to just do a C-section on everybody. It's a growing crisis, with some C-section rates at individual hospitals as high as 68%. Clearly, if someone does not step in and stop the trend, we will soon have C-section rates of 100%.

The third part of the problem is the insurance companies, because they are part of the establishment. When the obstetricians who give advice to the insurance companies say that home birth is dangerous or that midwives are not as safe as doctors, the CEOs of the insurance companies believe them.

There's no reason why they should look into it themselves; they get paid no matter who does the deliveries. The obstetricians are giving their opinion not on evidence-based findings, but because they see midwives as competition and an increased liability. Bottom line: doctors are the ones who have to do the surgery if something goes wrong. Therefore, many would rather do the surgery first instead of giving birth a chance.

The fourth problem is the dumbing down of the entire OB profession by losing the art of a breech delivery. The skills of delivering breech babies are no longer being taught in OB residencies.

Up until the year 2000, a woman carrying a breech baby at term had two choices: she could have a breech vaginal delivery or a breech cesarean delivery. In 2001, the vaginal breech delivery option disappeared almost entirely.

Approximately 4% of pregnancies end up in the breech presentation at full term. The United States has almost 4 million births per year, so now 160,000 women may be forced to accept a C-section as their only delivery option.

In reality, the option for vaginal breech birth was slowly being phased out in the late 1990s. Women were told that the baby's head could get stuck and then become asphyxiated and they would be a fool to ever have a breech delivery, but that is far from the truth. Breech vaginal deliveries are much safer than anyone would imagine.

The reason why vaginal breech deliveries are no longer part of the mainstream knowledge base of obstetricians is because of a single study called *The Term Breech Trial*, published in October 2000 in *The Lancet Public Health Journal.* It was not revealed until a few years later that the study had many flaws.

It initially showed that the outcomes for breech delivery were worse by vaginal birth than C-section, which in 2001 led the American College Of OB/GYN (ACOG) to publish a position paper in their annual Compendium stating that unless a breech baby is falling out of the vagina upon arrival to the hospital, the woman should have an emergent C-section. Not long after, the majority of North American doctors stopped doing breech vaginal deliveries because if they didn't stop, they would be going against the newly established community standards.

Before we knew it, breech deliveries died out in residency programs and economic incentives for doctors leaned towards doing sections. Unfortunately, it wasn't until a few years later that Dr. M. Glezerman, a researcher from Israel, took a critical look at the Term Breech Trial study and found that it included unplanned breech deliveries, premature breech deliveries, and babies with congenital anomalies, all of which had skewed the results in favor of section.

The results were corrected to not include these factors, but the damage was done. Still, to Dr. Glezerman's credit, he was one of the first to admit that a mistake was made. The following conclusions were stated in the documentary film *Heads Up: The Disappearing Art of Vaginal Breech Birth.*

*"**Conclusion:** Planned delivery is NOT associated with a reduction in risk of death or neurodevelopmental delay in children at 2 years of age."*
~ DEPARTMENT OF PEDIATRICS
TORONTO, ONTARIO, CANADA, 2004

*"**Conclusion:** The original term breech trial recommendations should be withdrawn."*
~ DR. M. GLEZERMAN, 2006

*"**Conclusion:** Elective section does NOT guarantee the improved outcome of the child, but may increase risks for the mother, compared to vaginal delivery."*
~ UNIVERSITY MEDICAL CENTER
GRONINGEN, THE NETHERLANDS 2007

By 2006, ACOG revised their recommendation by saying, "cesarean breech delivery will be the preferred mode for most physicians because of the diminishing expertise in vaginal breech delivery." Even if a doctor was trained to deliver breeches vaginally; they opt to do C-sections to avoid the liability of doing a vaginal breech delivery. Therefore, women are not given a choice.

There are a dismaying number of women out there who have spontaneously gone into rapid active labor with the baby in breech presentation and, upon arrival to the hospital, were forced to keep their legs together while their baby's butt was already in the vagina about to deliver.

In this condition, these women were rapidly taken to the OR, separated from their family, and given general anesthesia to have a rapid section. This whole scenario is completely unsafe for both the mother and child, but it has become the norm.

Even if a woman finds a doctor willing to do a vaginal breech delivery, they are often faced with the disclaimer, "I'll do it, but I really don't want to because it's not of the normal community standards and therefore it is not well supported among my peers." This increases the anxiety on the part of the practitioner and becomes one of the driving forces why breech vaginal deliveries are rarely done.

There are some risks in having a vaginal breech delivery, but the risk is minimal if protocols are followed. But first you must be taught these protocols, and because they are no longer a standard at the residency level, the art will soon be lost.

All this makes everyone around the laboring breech woman nervous and anxious. She then picks up on this anxious environment, making it very challenging for her to remain calm. This anxiety and nervousness may cause her cervix to tighten and not relax and dilate.

Women with breech-presenting babies find themselves in a stressful pregnancy and birth journey when it doesn't have to be that way. The conversations with most practitioners are usually one-way and do not include options.

Sometimes an External Cephalic Version (ECV) is offered, but that is becoming less common. This is a procedure that takes place in a hospital with the OR ready to go; doctors attempt to manually rotate the baby to a head-down position from outside the mother's abdomen.

An ECV is successful about 40 to 50% of the time, and if successful, is usually followed immediately with induction of labor to avoid the chance the baby will go back into a breech presentation. If the procedure fails, women are left feeling stressed, isolated, selfish, and anxious, when it has nothing to do with any added risk factors of medical problems with the mom or baby. All of this strife is due to a lack of access to information and choices.

In the documentary Heads Up, Homeland actress Morena Baccarin was one of several women followed in their quest for a breech vaginal birth.

"Like many women, the realization that her baby is breech forces Morena to face difficult decisions in the final weeks of her pregnancy. After exhaustive research Morena decides to plan for a vaginal breech birth with Dr. Wu. Several hours after this interview Morena went into labor. Within hours of arriving at the hospital, Morena is fully dilated and ready to deliver her baby. It is not uncommon for babies in a complete breech position to emerge feet first. After careful examination and evaluation, Dr. Wu determines it's safe to continue. Julius Setta Chick was born just after 5:00am, 7 pounds 15.4 ounces feet first."

–HEADS UP

"It's important for me that people learn about breech options because it doesn't have to be such a taboo, it doesn't have to be anxiety producing, it doesn't have to be a negative experience, it really truly is a miracle that little person came out of me and especially the way he did, it was the most profound love I've ever felt in my entire life. It's really sad to think that vaginal breech cannot be an option anymore and I think that is where we are headed. It was just seen as a regular birth with Dr. Wu and that's what you don't get with other doctors."

–MORENA BACCARIN

ACTOR, HOMELAND

Dr. Ronald Wu's success rate is 90% – only one out of ten of his breech deliveries end up in a C-section. Now when you compare that to the fact that one in three women in the US will have a C-section, you see how amazing those numbers are.

Most women don't get the information that their doctor does not do vaginal breech deliveries until they are well into their third trimester at about 37 weeks – and that is if they are lucky to have even that much advance notice.

In some cases, like mine, the baby turns at the last moment before labor and surprise, there you are breech and ready to push but no one is around who is well-trained. Still, knowing in advance that you have a breech baby isn't much better, because here in South Florida, for example, it is really hard to find a new doctor that will take over your care late in the pregnancy, let alone be willing to do a breech vaginal delivery.

Some hospitals have as high as a 68% C-section rate even if the baby is head down. Sadly, I see this as many doctors being driven by economics and convenience, and practicing defensive medicine instead of the art of medicine.

The dilemma of delivering natural obstetrical care to women needs to start changing on the grass roots level. First, each woman must learn that she has choices – and then have the courage to ask for what she wants.

Granted, home births and breech births may not be for everyone. But informed decision-making is. The more we give up our right to decide what is best for us, the more the decision will be made for us – and not necessarily for our best benefit.

We are taught to trust in modern medicine and procedures. Obstetricians are well-educated, and when they are needed they are extremely helpful. But a trained surgeon is not the right practitioner to be talking to about natural childbirth. In fact, in many regions there are midwives that continue to practice and teach vaginal breech deliveries.

It's time to bring back the art of delivering breech babies *and* the art of natural birth back to OB residency programs. The best way is to bring the honor and skills of midwifery care into the hospitals involved in teaching these residents. If we want our birth options to be protected, we need to let our desires be known.

Barriers to Options of OB Healthcare Providers

I've seen many times that most doctors will support midwives when they see it as lightening their work load and increasing their revenue at the same time. Less work and more money have to go hand in hand, or else the midwife will find herself out of a job.

Most doctors do not hire a midwife to provide better care, instead they want a mini-me, mid-level practitioner to do normal cases, so they can spend more time doing GYN surgery. You might ask, well why don't midwives just start their own practice? Well, in some states that's allowed, while in other states it's not.

Some states allow Certified Professional Midwives (CPM) or Licensed Midwife (LM) to have their own practice while they have laws that deny Certified Nurse Midwives (CNM) to have their own practice. An example is Florida, for a little while LM were allowed to do home births and have their own practice while CNMs were denied this because the CNM fell under the Nursing Practice Act of the state. It's fucked up! Meanwhile, states like Oregon, you can deliver a baby if you are a chiropractor! The laws keep changing and now CNM's can have their own practice in Florida.

It gets very muddy when you start to look at the disparity of who gets to be a "real" independent practitioner and whether insurance will reimburse them for their services. Yikes…. I guess I am trying to say is that you should research the laws and norms of your state and communities if you are looking for an alternative birth outside the hospital system. This is particularly crucial if you live in an area where the local hospitals ban VBACs.

In the movie, *The Business of Being Born*, Marsen Wagner MD, former Director of Women's and Children's Health for the World Health Organization (WHO), stated, *"If I am lecturing to a room full of obstetricians and I put the word home and the word birth together in the same sentence, there is just hysteria in the room. And then what I always do is just say, 'Ok, ok, I want everyone in this room who has ever attended a home birth raise your hand.' Nobody, they have never seen a home birth. So, I say, 'You are all like the geographers, who are trying to describe a country they have never been to, because they are too afraid to go there.'"*

If you look at the seven countries that have at least 400,000 births per year, the United States has the highest infant mortality of them all. One argument that is made for this is that we have different woman, a population that is less homogeneous and that causes higher risk scenarios, but blaming the diversity of women is false. It's really about how we treat care in the United States, but no one wants to admit that the healthcare system is failing women.

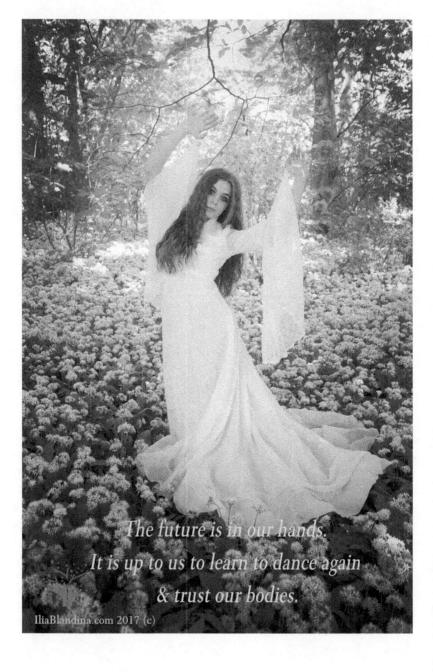

The future is in our hands.
It is up to us to learn to dance again
& trust our bodies.

CHAPTER 10

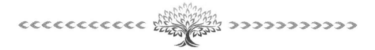

Our Birth Future

"You take your life in your own hands, and what happens?
A terrible thing: no one to blame."

~ ERICA JONG

The Importance of Taking Responsibility for Your Birth

W omen have been told for nearly a century that they are not responsible for their own birth process. This is so wrong! The established medical profession has convinced the majority of women that they don't know how to give birth.

Many healthcare providers feel that there is no stopping technology, so if you are going to have advances, you might as well use them to get the best outcome. But even J.W. Williams, the author of *Williams Obstetrics*, put it this way:

> *"Unfortunately, history shows that advances in the practice*
> *of medicine and surgery are rarely attained in a thoroughly*
> *rational manner, but that a period of undue enthusiasm,*
> *or even of almost reckless abuse, usually precedes the*
> *establishment of the actual value of a given procedure."*
> ~ JOHN WHITRIDGE WILLIAMS
> PIONEER OF ACADEMIC OBSTETRICS

When he wrote this, a C-section was an emergency operation, done only under the direst circumstances. He did note that even back then, C-sections were on the rise.

We should be asking ourselves: is avoiding VBACs an improvement, or are we making things worse? My opinion is we are making things worse, and if we don't take hold of this problem we may lose normal birth altogether.

For the average low-risk woman, it's overkill going to a doctor. It's just too much. The doctor is not really excited about things when they are normal. Midwives have done a better job at the normal deliveries than obstetricians; in many cases, they are the ones teaching residents how to do a normal delivery. For the most part obstetricians are taught to search for pathology first and foremost, so very often they see pathology where there is none.

The Midwifery Model Works for Birth

The midwifery model of care works in all the other countries. And when you look at the amount of money the United States spends versus the outcomes we get, it's awful. There are countries that spend a third of what we have and have lower infant mortality.

More interventions do not mean better healthcare; in fact, less intervention in the birth process is better healthcare. For example, the

Netherlands loses fewer women and babies than we do, and **one third** of their births are planned home births.

Ina May Gaskin, a midwife who started doing home births in 1970, reported having a 1.7% C-section rate from 1970 to 2010 out of a total of 2844 women accepted into care. That translated into a total of 50 C-sections. Her success rate for VBACs in the same time frame was 96.8%. This is what she says about the climb of the US C-section rates:

"So when I started only 5% of the women in the US had cesarean sections. Ten years past and it was up to about one woman in four. I couldn't believe it. And we didn't need, in our group, the first C-section until birth number 187. So we were going the other way, from the rest of the country. And we were doing that safely. So that told me something about the pelvis of the American woman is just quite fine, thank you very much, and we didn't have another C-section until birth number 324."

~ INA MAY GASKIN, CPM

EXECUTIVE DIRECTOR OF THE FARM BIRTH CENTER

The United States spends twice as much per birth than any other country in the world and yet our maternal and neonatal mortality is one of the worst in the world. Everywhere else in the world, if you look at Great Britain, France, Germany, Scandinavia, Australia, New Zealand, Japan, all the highly-developed countries where they are losing fewer women and fewer babies around the time of birth, you see midwives attending 70 or 80% of the births.

Doctors are only there to take care of the small percentages that develop the complications. That is the proven system everywhere in the world and yet the United States remains standing alone by keeping midwives out of the hospital as the standard of care.

We know that there is serious increase in minimal neurological problems in children and in attention deficit disorders, in autism; all of these things are increasing at the same period of time that we are increasing all these obstetric interventions in the US. Maybe, we don't really know this, but during the next few years will we discover to our horror that what happens at birth is very important to the future development of our children?

"If there's even a 1% chance of a terrorist act occurring, we must treat that as if it were a certainty. [From the book The One Percent Doctrine by Ron Suskind] This is a perfect description of the philosophy of contemporary maternity care, because when you set up a system that focuses on the 1% of problems that might occur you undermine the care of the 99% of mothers who don't need those services."

~ EUGENE R. DECLERCQ PHD

PROFESSOR OF MATERNAL CHILD HEALTH, BOSTON UNIVERSITY SCHOOL OF PUBLIC HEALTH.

I found this to be true in my own practice. During an interview with a prospective physician employer, I asked him if the risk of becoming pregnant after a bilateral tubal ligation is 1 chance out of 100 and the risk of uterine rupture is much less (1 chance in 1146), then why do you tell women that a tubal ligation is a permanent birth control option? In reality they have a higher chance of becoming pregnant after that procedure than they do of having a uterine rupture, which is the main argument for **not** having a VBAC.

His answer: "Well you can control one option, but you can't control the other." Think about that, he just admitted that because they as physicians can control what they offer, they will. It has nothing to do with what is better for you or your baby or informed consent.

The VBAC Pendulum

Historically, up until the mid-1970s, VBACs were not done. In fact, there was an old saying, "Once a C-section, always a C-section." This was in all the text books of the time but most uterine incisions were vertical and that type of incision increased the risk of uterine rupture during pregnancy as well as in labor. The uterine incisions were changed to horizontal which prevents uterine rupture in pregnancy and labor. Then, they started to question: Is it really that dangerous to have a VBAC?

By the early 1980s, VBAC became very popular and eventually were mandated. Even insurance companies who represent the women insisted that they should have a trial of labor. Of course, part of that was driven by economics. It is less expensive to have a vaginal birth than to have a C-section.

By the 1990s, the rate of VBAC increased to 28%. In contrast, today only 8% of women attempt a VBAC and out of that 8%, about 75% are successful, which means that 92% of women have a second cesarean. So the pendulum has swung back to "Once a C-section, always a C-section" birth philosophy.

When women were mandated to have VBACs instead of letting them just go into labor on their own, many were induced or augmented. This led to more complications during a trial of labor. Again, in their enthusiasm for VBACs, they forgot to trust in the woman's body.

After many VBACs they started to look at the data and found that uterine rupture was a low risk if women went into labor on their own. The risk of a bad outcome only increased if aggressive interventions were used to make a VBAC happen. This led the American College of OB/

GYN (ACOG) to keep changing their recommendations to reflect an increasingly more conservative position regarding VBACs because even though the risks are low, they felt it was safer to just do the surgery. It's not until recently, that we have found that as the C-section rate has climbed so has maternal and fetal poor outcomes.

The problem became that despite ACOG being very clear on their stance that a woman's choice should be held in the highest regard and that she has a right to control her own body, they also mandated all of these VBAC rules. ACOG also helped fan the flame regarding whether out-of-hospital birth was safe at all. This has led the obstetric community to limit a woman's options in order to prevent potential bad outcomes.

A study was done that asked women whether or not they would choose a VBAC. Only half were interested in exercising that option. It's quite possible this was partly due to women having been repeatedly told for the last decade that VBACs are not safe. Over time, repeat C-sections are what have been reinforced instead of having an informed choice.

During what is called informed consent, if you happen to find a doctor willing to do a VBAC, it usually goes like this:

"If you choose to have a VBAC, you must understand that you have a 1 in 200 chance that your uterus will rupture and that it may be catastrophic to you and your baby. This means you or your baby may die or survive and be in a vegetative state with poor quality of life. Even if you decide to have your VBAC in the hospital where an obstetrician and anesthesiologist are readily available, you may still suffer a catastrophic outcome. Are you still interested in having a VBAC?"

No lie, this is what is said, and this is what was said to me. Now, I want you to take in the whole picture. There I was with my husband, sitting in my doctor's office in 2003, receiving our "informed consent" talk. Both my husband and I are well-educated. He has a master's degree in education; I am a Certified Nurse Midwife, with years of obstetric experience.

I turned to my husband and said, "Gary, so what that means is, I might die and the baby might die, and everything may go to hell in a hand basket, are you okay with that?" He said, "Whatever you want to do, I'm with you." I turned to the doctor and said, "We are informed, I will do a VBAC."

You may be asking yourself, how can she be so "balls to the wall" about this? Does she really want to take that risk? Here is what I know as a midwife: The fact is, the chance of a uterine rupture is about 0.5% (or a 1 in 200 chance). And most of those ruptures aren't even discovered until the woman is either having another C-section or even later in their life, when they might have some kind of abdominal surgery and the surgeon inadvertently finds a tear in the uterus which then qualifies as a uterine rupture.

In actuality, the chance of a *catastrophic* uterine rupture is 1 in 2000 and by catastrophic, I mean the mother dies, the baby dies, or the baby suffers severe brain damage. **And a uterine rupture can even happen if it's your first baby.**

In contrast, consider **amniocentesis, a risk that women are willing to take every day that has a 1 in 200 or 1 in 400 chance of killing their baby.** So basically, a bleak picture of VBAC is painted during the "informed consent" process, but an amniocentesis, with its higher risk of a poor outcome, is ok and of course is offered to many women who are pregnant for possibly their last or only chance at having a baby.

What also doesn't get mentioned is the considerable increased risks of a repeat C-section, especially for women having their third or fourth repeat surgery. Risks of repeat C-sections are as follows:

- Higher risk of hysterectomy
- Increased risk of maternal mortality
- Increased risk of infection and wound complications
- Increased hospital stay

- Increased risk of damage to internal organs (bowel, bladder, ureteral injuries)
- Increased risk of bowel obstruction
- Increased risk of blood clots
- Increased risk of prolonged separation from baby and interruption in bonding
- Increased risk of unsuccessful breastfeeding
- Long-term development of adhesions (internal scar tissue) that lead to chronic pelvic pain
- Increased risk of bleeding requiring blood transfusion
- Placental abnormalities
- Placenta previa (the placenta attaches in front of the cervical opening)
- Placenta accreta or placenta percreta (both of these are varying degrees of the placenta attaching itself to include the uterine muscle wall).
- These placental abnormalities are life threatening situations that have increased 30-fold in the last 30 years alongside of the increase in C-section.

Of course, I knew all these things because I am in the medical community. These risks aren't discussed outside the medical community because if that's what you are up against, the theory goes, why even risk getting pregnant?

The point of all of this is not to scare you. It is to let you know that anyone can throw the numbers either way, but only you can decide what is right for you and your family. You have to do your own research and find a provider that is open to a VBAC who will give you unbiased consultation.

In my situation, I knew I was fine. I had two previous vaginal births, one C-section because the doctor didn't know how to do a breech delivery (and that was him saying that, not me), and then I was pregnant for the last time. I was 41 years old, and no, I did not have an amniocentesis. Yes, a VBAC was going to be ok.

I was not interested in turning my birth into major abdominal surgery and I knew I could do it. But still the supposed informed consent process is definitely framed in a way that would scare most of the general public, and that's why there has been an increase in the C-section rate.

As a midwife, I also know the ideal birth scenario is when you surround yourself with nurturing and supportive people and an environment you can control. You have the complete support of your partner. You have a midwife and a doula on your team. You are surrounded by the energy of love.

Unfortunately, in a VBAC situation, you often have the complete opposite. You may not be able to find a practitioner willing to do a VBAC or a hospital willing to do a VBAC. Even if either is willing, everyone is approaching it from a fear-based perspective, all waiting and watching for the worst-case scenario to happen.

The irony is that in each case, all you are trying to do is have a normal vaginal birth, and it really shouldn't be so controversial. I chose to have my baby at home because I didn't want all that fear drama in my birth journey, and I knew it was the safest place to be to have the least amount of intervention possible.

I knew my odds of success were much better at home. It's unfortunate that many women who want a VBAC have to fight and struggle to fulfill their choice and many times are not given all of the information needed to have an informed consent.

How VBACs Will Protect Our Future

The future of our health depends on the resurgence of VBAC becoming the norm again. There is emerging research suggesting that our immune system and therefore our health as adults are connected to how we are born.

First, research suggests that a small number of bacteria may be present in the placenta and in the womb, but the true seeding of our microbiome (the microorganisms in a particular environment, including the body) travels from the mother to the baby via the birth canal during birth.

Vaginal birth is the baby's first introduction to the world of bacteria that we live in. The process of vaginal birth becomes the foundation of our microbiome and immune system for the rest of our life.

Why is this important? Studies have shown that compared to tribes who are still living undisturbed by modern life, we have lost a third of our ancient microbes, and this change in the ancient microbiome that has protected us from many diseases is degrading.

This is in part due to 70 years of overuse of antibiotics – and you can't do surgery without using antibiotics. So with the advent of a whole generation of increased number of C-sections, the use of antibiotics (which are needed for every C-section) and bypassing the natural seeding of our microbiome by bypassing vaginal birth all causes our micro-diversity to diminish.

Rodney Dietert, professor of Immunotoxicology at Cornell University, believes that the microscopic process that happens during vaginal childbirth is critical for our future health. His hypothesis is called "The Complete Self," and it offers the idea that we are intended to be a majority microbial from the beginning of life at birth. When we are healthy, we are 90% microbial, and these good microbes are the foundation of our immune system because they prevent bad microbes from growing.

As humans, we are meant to be a micro-universe mirroring the cosmos.

The first major seeding of our microbiome is when the baby comes down the birth canal during vaginal birth. A healthy vagina has 300 to 400 microbes that provide the security for us by helping to set up our immune system at birth.

The next stage of microscopic transfer of microbes happens during skin-to-skin with the mother. This allows for the transfer of skin bacteria from the mother to the baby and is important for hormonal balance as well.

The natural habitat for the baby is to stay with the mother. When all of this is allowed to occur, oxytocin (the love hormone) is released and cortisol (the stress hormone) goes down.

It's an absolutely critical time, and this moment will never happen again with such intricate natural design. The body heat from mom regulates the baby's temperature; the baby will stay calm and naturally seek the mother's breast.

This is also a time when the mother and father will first look into the baby's eyes and create the first stage of falling in love, which actually sets a template for the future in life.

Breastfeeding is, as we all know, the best option, and the baby needs it for several reasons. First, the mother provides certain immune hormones that protect the baby. They include anti-inflammatory hormones, antibodies against diseases, more microbes, and oligosaccharide sugars.

These sugars cannot be digested by the baby, but they are present in breast milk to feed the good bacteria that were just seeded during vaginal birth and help the good microbes grow in the baby's gut. This helps the baby's developing immune system learn which bacteria are good ones, which should be tolerated, and which bacteria are bad and should be attacked.

So, if any of these steps are interrupted, as in the case of the increasing rate of C-sections, and the baby does not pass through the birth canal, this is what happens:

- The baby will bypass the mother's bacteria.
- The baby will have been exposed to antibiotics needed for the surgery.
- There may be problems breastfeeding.
- The baby will not be exposed to the skin-to-skin transfer of bacteria from the mother.
- The baby may potentially be exposed to other sources of bacteria from the hospital prior to establishing its health microbiome from mom.

Also, the squeezing effect of passing through the vagina does not occur during a C-section, and the baby does not effectively clear its lungs of the fluid from intrauterine life on its own. The latest research is also linking the seeding of the baby's microbiome with the development of other tissues, including the brain.

Because we now know that the diversity of the microbes in the gut affect the development of the brain and nervous tissue, a number of neural behavioral disorders have been linked with the microbes not being diverse enough. It is thought that the by-products that are produced by a diverse microbiome in the gut help the growth and development of the brain via transfer through the vagus nerve. If the diversity of the microbes in the baby's gut isn't seeded well at birth, this may lead to changes in the brain in ways that produce behavioral alterations.

In the last 20 to 30 years, we have seen a dramatic increase in asthma, Type 1 diabetes, celiac disease, and childhood obesity, all alongside the increased rates of C-section. We know that C-sections do not allow the baby to be seeded with the mother's microbes; this in turn interferes with the development of the immune system and is associated with changes in metabolism.

We now know that it is immune dysfunction and metabolic changes that contribute to these diseases. So, the questions are, could we be producing a generation of children who are missing vital bacteria? And could that be passed down to future generations? What is not known is what the consequences of this might be for humanity.

The Ultimate Goal for Birth

This does not mean we should stop doing C-sections altogether, but we need to find ways to deal with the problem when a C-section is needed. One turning point is to decrease the C-section rate by not doing elective C-sections and whenever possible promoting trial of labor for women who have had prior C-sections.

Changing the birth paradigm back towards natural support of VBAC will decrease the overall cesarean section rates. By "natural support of VBAC," I mean as practitioners relearn to trust in women's bodies and as women learn how to trust their own bodies.

Doing this is a matter of managing our personal fears and doubts so that we can give birth a chance. This also needs to involve truthful informed consent instead of twisting the facts to benefit the healthcare system by instilling fear in expectant mothers and fathers.

If a mother must have a C-section, there are ways being developed that she can still promote the seeding of the baby's microbiome. There is an idea of using vaginal swabs prepared before delivery using sterile gauze soaked in sterile saline, folded into a fan pattern, and placed in the vagina for an hour before birth. Then it is removed and placed into a sterile container.

After the birth by C-section, the gauze with mom's vaginal microbes is used to wipe the inside of the baby's mouth, face, and body, simulating the normal seeding as if born via the birth canal. The next step is to have skin-to-skin contact immediately after birth if at all possible, and to breastfeed for longer than a year, optimally until the baby weans itself.

The Economic Factors

The health insurance companies for mothers all know that a vaginal birth – and therefore a VBAC – is more cost-effective than a C-section. The problem lies with the insurance companies that provide malpractice coverage. Many do not cover the practitioner for doing a VBAC, or, if they do cover VBAC, then the insurance premium is too high and it forces practitioners to not offer VBACs because they can't afford the insurance. In effect, the insurance companies are then controlling medical practice by creating an economic penalty for providing the service. It's crazy!

Meanwhile, hospitals have gotten used to the higher revenue they make by creating a "once a C-section, always a C-section" environment. First, they make more money by doing C-sections, because it is major abdominal surgery and requires the entire infrastructure of major surgery, including anesthesia, plus many hospitals have adopted the policy that all C-section babies have to stay in the NICU for the first four hours of life! This also brings in more money. Ka-ching!

The protocols are different from hospital to hospital; they are not regulated across the board on a state-wide or national level in regard to labor and delivery. Evidence-based medicine is now exactly the opposite. It is showing that women are better off not having a repeat C-section, but the way the system is set up now, we are forcing women to have a surgery that carries more risk than if you let them labor and have a successful VBAC.

Many hospitals at the moment do not want to take the risk of VBAC, because it's all risk and very little monetary reward for them despite the fact that ACOG recently stated that for women who delivered vaginally with a successful VBAC, the risk of complications are fewer than if they have an elective repeat C-section.

The big push should be that women have the correct informed consent and informed refusal. They have to have all of the information presented in a non-biased way. Woman also need to be in control of their birth process and they have to be given choices to do what they feel is comfortable and what feels most optimal for themselves.

On the other hand, *"with great power comes great responsibility."* If people are given the choices and different options for the birth of their children, they also have to accept the responsibility for the choices they make. In other words, if something goes wrong, don't blame it on the choices you made in good faith about having an alternative birth option. There are no choices without risk; this is true in all aspects of life. After you decide how best to give birth, believe in yourself and what feels true for you.

In 2010, ACOG revised their Practice Bulletin, giving women and their practitioners more flexibility to decide what is the best way to give birth. ACOG stated that more women should be considered appropriate VBAC candidates, including women with two previous C-sections, women carrying twins, and women with unknown uterine scars from a previous surgical procedure.

*****

The Ultimate Birth Truth Statements

Follow these steps to write your ultimate birth truth statements regarding your birth journey. First, come up with five statements describing your birth. They must be affirmative and in present tense.

A few examples are:

- I am having regular contractions.
- I trust my body and it knows what to do. I am pushing
- My baby is being born vaginally.

Next to those five statements, list five positive impacts on your life from these events and describe an associated positive emotion. You will end up with three columns of information. It will look something like this:

I am having regular contractions	My labor started on its own	I feel calm
I trust my body	I have more confidence	I feel safe
My body knows what to do in labor	I have freedom to move while in labor	I feel empowered
I am pushing very well	I have energy	I feel strong
My baby is being born vaginally	My recovery is effortless	I feel joyful
My partner is by my side	I am secure	I feel love and happiness

Feel free to substitute your own words. Now you give thanks to the Creator for bringing this to you. Write out all the elements in sentences:

- I am thankful that I feel calm because my labor has started on its own and I am having regular contractions.
- I am thankful that I feel safe because I have more confidence and I trust my body.
- I am thankful that I feel empowered because I have the freedom to move while in labor and my body knows what to do in labor.
- I am thankful that I feel strong because I have energy and I am pushing very well.
- I am thankful that I feel joy because my recovery is effortless and my baby is born vaginally.

- I am thankful that I feel love and happiness because I am secure and my partner is by my side.

Each day, use these statements to tap with as described in Chapter 7. If any negative thoughts or doubts come into your mind while you are tapping, write them down in your journal and use the set-up statement from Chapter 7.

- "Even though I thought [blank] and it makes me feel [blank], I deeply and completely accept myself."

Remember to get a SUDs level before you start tapping. You need to tap on anything that comes up until the negative emotions are neutralized. Change the elements in the table and the full statements as needed.

One more step. I want you to find the love letter you wrote to yourself at the end of Chapter 1 and read it. How does it compare to your Ultimate Birth Truth Statements? Look to see if you were in alignment at the beginning of this book or focusing on all the negative things that may happen. All of this information and insight will serve you, because you can use tapping to help clear the way to your best birth journey. All is well.

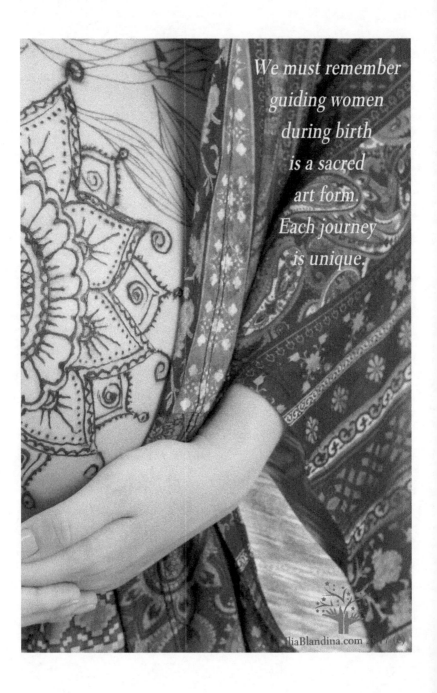

We must remember
guiding women
during birth
is a sacred
art form.
Each journey
is unique.

IliaBlandina.com

CONCLUSION

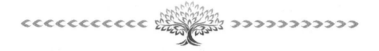

*"There came a time when the risk to remain tight in the bud
was more painful than the risk it took to blossom."*
~ ANAIS NIN

Reflecting on My Birth Journeys as Midwife and Client

et's look at our journey. Retrospectively, first and foremost, I have to apologize. I have been part of the system as a CNM that is breaking the heart of women – and yet I have also been part of the movement that empowers women as a client.

It has not been easy to be a midwife in South Florida. It's driven by a "good old boy" system of a "what can you do for me?" attitude on the part of the medical community. How many patients can you see? How many deliveries can you do a month? I once attended 11 births in less than 16 hours; it almost killed me. But, I couldn't complain. I had to suck it up.

On the other side of the coin, when it came to me, my body, my baby, there was no way in hell I wanted to be in the hospital. Yes, the hospital was handy when I had to transfer from a birth center for my first and second pregnancies, but then my third pregnancy that was a planned hospital birth with a midwife ended in a C-section because the doctor on call was of the generation that does not know how to do a normal breech delivery.

For my fourth and final birth, I had to run away. I had to go underground. I knew I could have a homebirth, but I still had to trick myself by telling myself, "Oh, I'm just preparing for a homebirth in case I go fast. My midwife friends will just come over and hang out. It will just be a gathering." Well, my work-around worked. I had my dream homebirth.

The Take-Away for You

What I want you to take away from all these concepts, ideas, and suggestions is that you don't have to have a "work-around" "psych-out" plan to make your dream birth happen. During the writing of this book, I went for my annual GYN exam. My practitioner and I use to practice midwifery together, so we've known each other for a long time.

She asked me, "Where are you practicing these days?" I said enthusiastically, "I'm helping women overcome their fears of having a VBAC." She replied, "Who's doing VBACs these days?" It was all I could do not to scream. I replied, "Well, obviously, it's hard to find someone in South Florida, but I intend to help the whole world." She has a great sense of humor and replied, "So you've got the whole world in your hands?" I said, "Sure!"

In reality, WE must all work together to Give Birth A Chance! I never want to hear the words, "Who's doing VBACs these days?" again. WE as women have to make a stand and take birth back.

Give Birth A Chance was written because I wanted to help STOP the pendulum of the high C-section rate in this country! It's been getting out of control and very few people are talking about what really is going on behind the scenes.

Because of fear-based thinking on both sides, the pregnant woman and the practitioner are both perpetuating the idea that having a C-section is the safest option around, when in reality, letting woman labor on their own and providing a supportive, safe, and empowering container is really the safest route. Our ability to birth has been truly on trial whether we knew it or not. And the judge's name is Fear.

I want to create an energetic space where my clients can find their strength to stand their ground. I want them to learn how to believe in themselves, despite any statistics or studies. I want them to have the power to choose their own journey.

The practitioners need healing as well, but first they need to see it from the perspective of their clients. As practitioners, we are here to guide our clients – not to scare them into doing what the book of policies and procedures says to do, or to make them fit into some prefabricated textbook mold of how labor should be.

We must come back to our humanity. We must come back to seeing birth as a normal process, not a train wreck waiting to happen. I wrote this book to find the women who need me to help them learn how to show up in a medical system that is scared out of its wits of being sued. In a system that treats women in labor like cattle. "Sorry, if you don't meet the labor curve, studies show you will be in danger, so we need to do a C-section or else."

The madness of fear needs to stop. But the first step is yours! The woman who shows up in labor or thinking she is in labor has to be confident in her body's ability to do the work of birth instead of being on trial for whether she can do the work.

My overall goal in writing this book was to open the door for women to have the conversation about what is possible in order to have the birth journey they desire.

Yes, you can give birth the way you want. At least, in the best possible positive state of mind: out of love, not fear.

Yes, there are ways you can get rid of those negative, fear-based thoughts in your head that keep floating up to the surface.

Yes, there is a way you can talk with friends and family members who are so willing to tell you their horrible birth stories under the guise of "I'm just trying to help."

Yes, yes, yes, you can do this.

The big secret is you have to learn how to do this on your own! Yes, you will have your supporters; I am one of them! But ultimately, you are alone during the birth process, no matter how many people are in the room holding your hand, rubbing your back, wiping your brow.

The Ultimate Moment in Birth

This ultimate moment of being in your body, by yourself, is what you really need to prepare for. The moment where you may feel lost, where doubt and fear start to creep in. This is what this book is about! It will give you the tools you need and the best foundation for giving birth your own way – the best and safest way possible.

This book is not for those who are on the fence about whether they want a VBAC. This book is for those who want to make a VBAC their reality and want a foundation of love to support their birth journey. So, read it, reread it, do the exercises. You won't be disappointed. And if you really want to increase your success of getting the birth you dreamed of, reach out to me at ilia@givebirthachance.com.

"... if you want to know where a woman's true power lies,
look to those primal experiences we've been taught to fear...
the very same experiences the culture has taught us to distance
ourselves from as much as possible, often by medicalizing

them so that we are barely conscious of them anymore. Labor
and birth rank right up there as experiences that put women
in touch with their feminine power...."
~ DR. CHRISTIANE NORTHRUP

"When the righteous cry for help,
the LORD hears and delivers them out of all their troubles."
~ PSALM 34:17

Since the writing of this book which was first published December 12, 2016, I am so happy to include that the American College of Obstetricians and Gynecologists (ACOG) COMMITTEE OPINION Number 687, February 2017 published *Approaches to Limit Intervention During Labor and Birth*.

Recommendations and Conclusions for women at term in spontaneous labor and the baby is head down, their management of labor may be individualized by including:

- The use of intermittent auscultation and nonpharmacologic methods of pain relief.
- Admission to hospital may be delayed during early labor.
- If a woman in early labor is admitted for pain or fatigue, nonpharmacologic techniques such as education, support, oral hydration, massage or water immersion should be used.
- Endorse the addition to regular nursing care, the use of doulas for continuous one-to-one emotional support is associated with improved outcomes for women in labor.
- Routine amniotomy should be avoided unless required to help monitor the baby.
- Use of the coping scale to best meet the needs of each woman.
- Frequent position changes.

- Each woman should be encouraged to use whatever technique she prefers and is most effective during pushing.
- When they are 10 centimeters dilated, and do not have an urge to push, let the woman rest for up to 2 hours unless there is an indication to hurry the birth.

There is much more detailed information in the 9-page document and I encourage you to read it for yourself.

https://www.acog.org/-/media/Committee-Opinions/Committee-on-Obstetric-Practice/co687.pdf

The bottom line is The Universe is hearing our plea to ***GIVE BIRTH A CHANCE!!!***

GIVE BIRTH A CHANCE MANIFESTO

- Transform all hospitals in the US to include the option of natural TOLAC
- All nurses working in labor and delivery units are Certified Nurse Midwives
- All obstetricians should only be consultants for labor and delivery units
- Medical malpractice reform laws to protect practitioners from litigation for circumstances beyond their control
- All labor units designed in a pentagon formation with a living atrium in the center including a grassy area that will allow laboring women to walk in an "outside," earthy environment
- Himalayan salt lamps in each room and on desks to absorb the positive ions in the electromagnetic field emissions of all the electronics on the unit
- Intermittent monitoring for all low-risk clients
- Doula care for every client, who will also function as a delivery assistant and who have Neonatal Resuscitation Protocol skills
- [Blank] Fill in the blank. What do you want to see change in our birth culture? Post your thoughts on www.facebook.com/givebirthachance/

"There are two basic motivating forces: fear and love. When we are afraid, we pull back from life. When we are in love, we open to all that life has to offer with passion, excitement, and acceptance. We need to learn to love ourselves first, in all our glory and our imperfections. If we cannot love ourselves, we cannot fully open to our ability to love others or our potential to create. Evolution and all hopes for a better world rest in the fearlessness and open-hearted vision of people who embrace life."

~ JOHN LENNON

Further Information

Books:

Back Labor No More!!: What Every Woman Should Know Before Labor by Janie McCoy King

The Biology of Belief: Unleashing the Power of Consciousness, Matter, & Miracles by Bruce H. Lipton, Ph. D.

Birth Matters: How What We Don't Know About Nature, Bodies, and Surgery Can Hurt Us by Ina May Gaskin

Birthing from Within: An Extra-Ordinary Guide to Childbirth Preparation by Pam England CNM MA & Rob Horowitz Ph. D.

Breaking the Habit of Being Yourself: How to Lose Your Mind and Create a New One by Dr. Joe Dispenza

Childbirth Without Fear: The Principles and Practice of Natural Childbirth by Grantly Dick-Read

Communing with the Spirit of your Unborn Child: A Practical Guide to Intimate Communication With Your Unborn or Infant Child by Dawson Church

The Divine Matrix: Bridging Time, Space, Miracles, and Belief by Gregg Braden

The EFT Manual: Emotional Freedom Techniques by Gary Craig

The Energy of Belief: Psychology's Power Tools to Focus Intention and Release Blocking Beliefs by Sheila Sidney Bender, PhD & Mary T. Sise, LCSW

The Gaia Effect by Kryon and Monika Muranyi

The Genie in your Genes: Epigenetic Medicine and the New Biology of Intention by Dawson Church

Heal Your Birth, Heal Your Life by Sharon King

The Human Akash: A discovery of the blueprint within by Kryon & Monika Muranyi

Immaculate Deception II: Myth, Magic and Birth by Suzanne Arms

Matrix Re-imprinting Using EFT: Rewrite Your Past, Transform Your Future by Karl Dawson & Sasha Allenby

Sacred Pregnancy: A Loving Guide and Journal for Expectant Moms by Anni Daulter

Spiritual Midwifery by Ina May Gaskin

Soul Shifts: Transformative Wisdom for Creating a Life of Authentic Awakening, Emotional Freedom & Practical Spirituality by Dr. Barbara DeAngelis

The Tapping Solution for Pain Relief: A Step-by-Step Guide to Reducing and Eliminating Chronic Pain by Nick Ortner

Transform Your Beliefs, Transform Your Life: EFT Tapping Using Matrix Re-imprinting by Karl Dawson & Kate Marillat

Women's Bodies, Women's Wisdom: Creating Physical and Emotional Health and Healing by Christiane Northrup, M.D.

You Are the Placebo: Making Your Mind Matter by Dr. Joe Dispenza

Orgasmic Birth: Your Guide to a Safe, Satisfying and Pleasurable Birth Experience by Elizabeth Davis and Debra Pascali-Bonaro

Nurturing Beginnings: A Guide to Postpartum Care for Doulas and Community Outreach Workers by Debra Pascali-Bonaro

Documentary Films:
The Business of Being Born (2008)

Spirit Space: A Journey into your Consciousness (2008)

The Living Matrix: A film on the new science of healing (2009)

Organic Birth: Birth is Natural (2010)

Orgasmic Birth: The Best Kept Secret (2012)

Freedom for Birth: A new documentary about human rights in childbirth (2012)

Birth Story: Ina May Gaskin and The Farm Midwives (2013)

Microbirth (2014)

Heads Up: The Disappearing Art of Vaginal Breech Delivery (2015)

Trial of Labor: A documentary about modern childbirth from the mother's perspective (2015)

Why Not Home? The Surprising Birth Choices of Doctors and Nurses (2016)

Acknowledgments

Inner Circle:

- Gary, my husband since 1981 and soul mate through many lifetimes, who has always been there for me at my highest and lowest moments. He has never given up on me, and I will never give up on him. He is the Father of the family and has patience beyond all measure, for all of this I am truly grateful to have created my life with him. His support in the birth of our family and this book is beyond measure. I cannot thank him enough.

- Alex, my first born. His name means "helper of mankind," and he has naturally grown into this meaning by studying Social Psychology at the PhD level. I remember him at 16 years of age, telling me during one of my mom rants about chores, *"Mom, it's okay; you just have to understand that we don't see the dirt you see. All you have to do is just tell us what you need and we will help clean it up. You don't have to be upset about it; you can choose to be happy."* Wow, my boys don't see dirt and I can choose to be happy! I'm still awed! Thank you, Alex, helper of mankind. His wife and best friend, Stephanie, is a jewel! Thank you for supporting Alex in his life purpose as I know he supports you.

- Andrew, my second son. His name means "strong man" and he has lived up to that name. He has shown me the importance of physical and mental strength and the determination to follow your dreams. Andrew, you have taught me how to have singularity of mind, and that life is just a play, filled with many roles, and you can choose the role you want to be in any circumstance. Thank you for being there for me through the hardest of times. His partner and best friend, Keith, is joy personified! Thank you for supporting both Andrew in his life purpose and our entire family.

- Aaron, my third son. His name means "enlightened one" and he has stepped into his name by revealing to us his God given gift of musicianship. As Henry Wadsworth Longfellow said, *"Music is the universal language of mankind,"* and so Aaron has also lived up to his name by giving us the gift of music as he interprets it. I remember him saying at dinner one evening, *"Jazz is like a blanket, when you listen to it the music covers you."* He was 12 years old. Thank you for the gift of music, a language that fills the space when words fail. To his partner and best friend, Danielle, thank you for being there for Aaron in his college and musical adventures.

- Adam, my fourth son, the baby! His name means "of the earth" and he has been my grounding gift from God. His hugs are like gold; he has been teaching me to take time to hug since he was a toddler! He still hugs me every day, even now at the dawn of his teen years!

- Tasha, Ranger, and Tessa, our furry companions throughout the years. Exemplifiers of unconditional love, protection, and friendship.

- All my sons' births have taught me how different birth can be. Each birth is a unique sacred event and the root of life's mysteries. Thank you for choosing me to be your Mother!

Origins:

- Mom, thank you. Without your foundation and advice, I would have never thought of being a nurse. You helped me get my first job at 16 in a hospital and taught me the importance of caring for people. In your memory, I continue the work beyond the physical aspects of bedside nursing and midwifery. It was from the miracles that happened around your passing that fueled the birth of this book and the study of mystical aspects of birth itself. RIP. October 24, 1931 to July 30, 2014.

- Dad, thank you for reading all those National Geographic books to me as a young girl. Through them, you helped lay the ground work for my scientific mind and enjoyment of seeking scientific evidence and truth. RIP. December 10, 1930 to August 30, 1985.

- Brother, Harry, my 180-degree reflection. Thank you for being the first born and for all your big brother advice, even when it wasn't well received by me. As time has passed, I see the wisdom. I remember when I was about six years old, and you were 15. I got a splinter in my bottom from scooting around on the wood floors; you were the only person I would let take it out. I knew even then that you would be able to do it without inflicting more pain. You will always be the best doctor in the world. Thank you to your longtime partner and wife, Leslie and my nephews and niece, Nathaniel, Ethan, and Annelise. The next generation is full of hope and vision!

- Stepfather, Luis, who was married to my Mom as long as my Dad, 25 years each. Thank you for being there for my Mom and my family. You were the only grandfather my children have known. Thank you for giving us many insights into life from stories of your childhood in Cuba to general sage wisdom at the dinner table. I remember your advice when my career kept changing employers, you said, "So what, your next job will always be better! Don't take it personally." RIP. November 13 (27), 1927 to May 8, 2011.

- Grandma Pumpkin, so named by Andrew! Thank you for raising such a wonderful son – my husband Gary – and his siblings Laura and Geri. All of you have been influential in my journey of writing this book. Coordinating fantastic family gatherings ranging from around the hearth to all the way in Alaska!

- Abuela Alejandrina, who I never met. She passed away before I was born, in 1954, but was said to have been the midwife and healer of my ancestral village in Puerto Rico. When I embarked on my journey as mother and midwife, my Uncle (her son and my Mom's brother) told me that she was my spirit guide. I asked him how he knew this. He asked me, "Don't you remember her name?" I replied, "No." You see I had my first baby, named him Alexander and had just entered into the study of nurse midwifery when my Uncle was chatting with me. Since that conversation, I know my Grandmother Spirit Guide has always been there at every birth giving me guidance and intuition. My ancestors are from the Taino Indians, Native Americans of the Caribbean. I thank all my ancestors for urging me to write this book and guiding me in all my research.

- José (Cheó) and Joann, my cousins. Thank you for mystical conversations and interpretation of the world. You planted the seed of the importance of our family purpose to make a difference in the world by helping people. Our bouillabaisse adventure will never be forgotten!

Colleagues:

- Ann Addison, CNM, was the labor nurse at Andrew's birth. We attended midwifery school together at the University of

Florida and she was the midwife at Aaron's birth. Thanks to you and Darrell for being with me and Gary during such great transitions. RIP. December 20, 1950 to October 30, 2014.

- Janice Heller, LM, my midwife with Adam's birth. A big thank you for holding the space for home birth in South Florida. Since 1978, she has dedicated her life's work to empowering women during pregnancy and birth. This has not been an easy task in Florida. Without her encouragement and guidance, I would not have had the beautiful empowering home birth of Adam. Thank you for being there for me and making my VBAC a normal birth experience. You opened my eyes to how birth really should be like.

- Fadwah Halaby, CNM, thank you for working with me at one of the busiest OB/GYN practices in the tri-county area. You taught me how to keep things natural in one of the most unnatural places for birth. Many blessings to your solo practice created to bring birth home again in South Florida.

Mentors:

- Alina Frank, thank you for teaching me EFT and Matrix Reimprinting. All our footsteps lead us together, and your influence in my personal growth goes beyond measure. Your divine entrance into my life was at the most pivotal time. You have introduced me to all of the following mentors and have continued to teach me the best methods of how to use EFT. There are no words, except a very heartfelt Thank You!

- Craig Weiner, DC, thank you for breaking down the scientific evidence of how EFT works. Your online class Tapping Out of Trauma is one of the most valuable classes I have taken beyond EFT itself. Thank you also for putting together an extensive collection of EFT-related research articles. You have made learning the science behind tapping easy! http://www.efttappingtraining.com/eft-research/

- Jenny Johnston, thank you for connecting me to my past lives through the development of your Quantum EFT methods. Also, a big thank you for introducing me to the teachings of Kryon.
- Angela Lauria, my agent at Difference Press. Thank you for being a birth junky. You gave me the confidence I needed to write this book and made it into a fun process. I look forward to our continued work together.
- Maggie McReynolds, my editor. Thank you for making sure my words made sense. I am so grateful for your guidance and expertise in managing the whole editing process. I could always count on you when my brain started to fog up.
- To the Morgan James Publishing team: Special thanks to David Hancock, CEO & Founder for believing in me and my message. To my Author Relations Manager, Tiffany Gibson, thanks for making the process seamless and easy. Many more thanks to everyone else, but especially Jim Howard, Bethany Marshall, and Nickcole Watkins.

Pioneers:
- Debra Pascali-Bonaro, thank you so much for writing the Foreword and creating the documentary that took the birth world by storm! *Orgasmic Birth: The Best Kept Secret*
- Nancy Wainer, CPM, the pioneering midwife who coined the term "VBAC". Thank you, Nancy, for reaching out to me for lunch while you were in Florida! What a wonderful surprise! Also, a big thank you for reading my manuscript and your endorsement of my mission with this book. Nancy is the author of the ground breaking book *Silent Knife: Cesarean Prevention*

and VBAC; Open Season: A Survival Guide for Natural Birth and the soon to be released *Birthquake: A Pre-and Post Childbirth Book for Strong Women and Women Who Want To Be Strong*

- Gary Craig, thank you for creating the process known as Emotional Freedom Techniques (EFT), it continues to change the world.

- Karl Dawson, thank you for creating the process known as Matrix Reimprinting and thereby joining the source field, quantum physics, and tapping all together. You have literally opened the door to time travel.

- Ina May Gaskin, the most famous midwife in the world. Thank you for reminding us how birth is so sacred and that a woman's body is not a lemon.

- Suzanne Arms, thank you for shining the light of how modern women have been steered away from believing in an empowered birth.

- Dr. Christiane Northrup, thank you for breaking free from the usual and customary understanding of women's healthcare needs.

- Dr. Barbara DeAngelis, thank you for keeping our appointment. As one of your students, I know you have been holding the energetic space for this book to be born.

- Dr. Bruce Lipton, thank you for thinking outside the box about our biology and proving that our genes do not predetermine our life.

- Greg Braden, thank you for searching for the answer to the big question, "Where did I come from and why am I here?"

- Dr. Joe Dispenza, thank you for making meditation easy and with lasting effects.

- Lee Carroll, thank you for saying yes to Kryon's channeling and for traveling the world to spread Kryon's teachings.

- David Wilcock, thank you for being one the most vigorous researchers of The Law of One: The Ra Material. Your Wisdom Teachings show on Gaia TV has been enlightening and given me a deeper understanding of Universal laws.

The Source Incarnate:

- Jesus Christ, thank you for always being with me and teaching me very early on that LOVE is the answer to all questions and frustrations of life. Without your loving words, we would be lost.
- Buddha, thank you for being the most quoted ascended master. Your words of wisdom are everywhere.

Thank you to all my Guides and Angels for helping me along my path to fulfill my life purpose through this book. Thank you to all the women who have given me the privilege of helping them during their birth journey.

ABOUT THE AUTHOR

Ilia Blandina CNM ARNP bestselling and award winning author of *Give Birth A Chance: How to Prepare for an Empowered VBAC.* Her first book was published for **Amazon Kindle** in December of 2016, quickly becoming an **international bestseller** on the first day of the book launch. Her book was featured as one of **The Best Pregnancy Books of 2016** by MotherRisingBirth.com. Ilia also was a featured **speaker at the ECO Baby Expo 2017**. She then became the recipient of **2017 International Book Award Finalist in the Health: Women's Health category.**

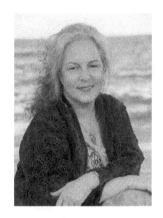

Ilia Blandina, CNM
EFT & Matrix Re-Imprinting Practitioner
Bestselling Author
Awaken Your Life Power, Inc.

Ilia has been practicing as a professional nurse midwife since 1994. She received her Bachelor of Science in Nursing with Honors from the University of Florida in 1985. After four years of nursing practice in the pediatric ICU & neonatal ICU she transferred to the Labor & Delivery unit at Shands Hospital in Gainesville Florida and continued her studies at the University of Florida, earning her Master of Science in Nursing degree by 1994.

She has varied practice experience ranging from rural to urban settings, helping to open a birth center in North Carolina to bringing more natural experiences to hospital birth settings. She has attended over 5000 births in her midwifery career.

She has held academic appointments as Clinical Instructor at Nova Southeastern University College of Nursing, University of Cincinnati College of Midwifery, and Frontier Nursing University College of Midwifery. In addition, she is a member of the American College of Nurse-Midwives (ACNM), AAMET International, DONA International, ACEP and APPPAH.

She is the founder of Awaken Your Life Power, Inc. (2011) a company devoted to inspiring people through their life journey and has created online communities for inspiration and educational support. She produced & hosted the Awaken Your Fertility Summit (2012). She has always been fascinated with alternative medicine and has studied herbal remedies, aromatherapy, metaphysics and Energy Psychology. Her study and certification in Emotional Freedom Techniques (EFT) and Matrix Re-Imprinting led her to develop the process of Childbirth With Grace™, a program that helps women shed their fears around birth. She shares her childbirth education knowledge online at www. IliaBlandina.com.

Through her years in midwifery practice she has found that overcoming your fears regarding your birth journey is the most key area of childbirth education especially if you have had a cesarean section and now want to plan for a vaginal birth after cesarean (VBAC).

Ilia has been married since 1981 to a wonderful husband and together they have been blessed with the birth of 4 boys, 2 vaginal births in a hospital that started out in a birth center, 1 cesarean section and 1 VBAC at home! Both as a midwife and mother she has walked the path of her clients which has created a deep passion for her work to help women become prepared for a VBAC and to teach C-section prevention techniques.

THANK YOU!

Thanks for reading this book! I'd love to hear from you about your birth stories and how you would love to Give Birth A Chance. Please message me or comment on Facebook at: www.facebook.com/givebirthachance/

Get your **FREE VBAC Tool Kit** at www.GiveBirthAChance.com The kit includes:

1. Birth Affirmation Self-Assessment Tool.
2. Four MP3 downloads for tapping sequences.
3. Four beautiful images to focus on.
4. Birth Journey Intentions: A list of needs starting with the statement, "I intend my birth journey to be safe and peaceful. With this in mind if safety allows, the following list is what I want to see happen during my birth journey."
5. Instructions on how to make an aromatherapy rice bag.
6. Ultimate Birth Truth Statement Worksheet.
7. Birth preparation exercises for your body and mind.

Free Strategy Session for an Empowered Birth:

Have you downloaded the Tool Kit and figured out you need help with preparing for an empowered birth? You can get started by filling out the form here:

https://www.givebirthachance.com/birthplan/
or email me at ilia@GiveBirthAChance.com
In all things, may you be at Peace and Blessed in your birth journey!
Ilia Blandina CNM

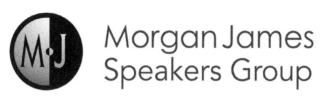

Morgan James
Speakers Group

↗ www.TheMorganJamesSpeakersGroup.com

We connect Morgan James published
authors with live and online events
and audiences who will benefit
from their expertise.

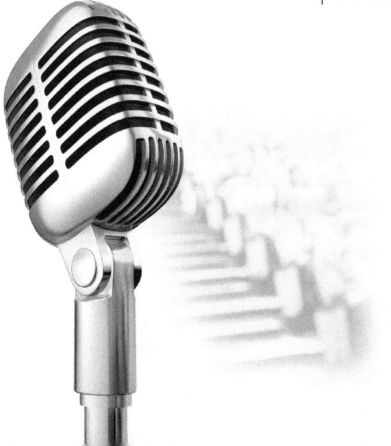

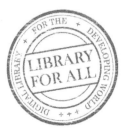

Morgan James makes all of our titles available
through the Library for All Charity Organization.

www.LibraryForAll.org

Printed in the USA
CPSIA information can be obtained
at www.ICGtesting.com
JSHW022330140824
68134JS00019B/1389

9 781683 505198